Taking Ca...

SENATOR
AVEL GORDLY

A
CAREGIVER RESOURCE
GUIDE

REV. DR. TYRONE W. WATERS,
D.D.,F.H.L.C.A.

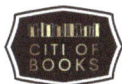

CITI OF
BOOKS

CITIOFBOOKS, INC.
3736 Eubank NE Suite A1
Albuquerque, NM 87111-3579
www.citiofbooks.com

Hotline: 1 (877) 389-2759
Fax: 1 (505) 930-7244

Ordering Information:
Quantity sales. Special discounts are available on
quantity purchases by corporations, associations, and
others. For details, contact the publisher at the address
above.

Printed in the United States of America.

ISBN-13: Paperback   979-8-89391-482-5
          eBook   979-8-89391-483-2

Library of Congress Control Number: 2024926362

TABLE OF CONTENTS

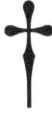

DEDICATION

I want to thank Elder Curtis Miller and Mother
Ivy Miller of Highland Christian Center for
teaching me to know what it means to be
a man and take care of my mother.

To my Mom Avel Gordly, I got this book project done
for you.

Blessing and Anointing.

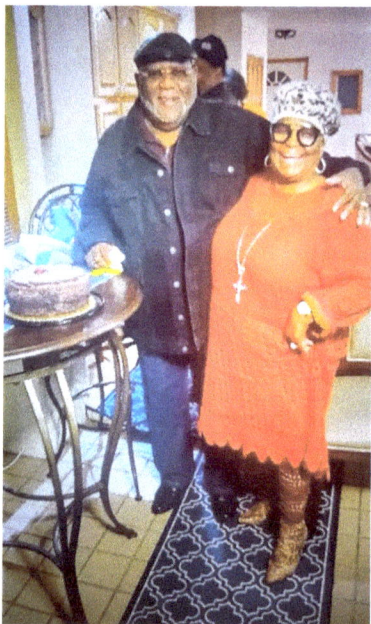

Elder Curtis Miller and Mother Ivy Miller

ACKNOWLEDGEMENT

Thank you my literary agent, Jason Collins, and Aiden Blake, fulfillment officer and to the rest of the COB team for helping me to get this project completed.

Caring and Coping

Everyone undoubtedly has a different experience with their loved one who has Alzheimer's. That's because every individual reacts differently to this difficult condition. Each person — and each family — has a unique way of coping with Alzheimer's and trying to minimize its disruption to family life.

Inevitably, though, Alzheimer's will disrupt your life. But the similarities among symptoms mean there are also similar ways of dealing with them. This *Caregiver's Support Kit*, through examples, case histories, and practical suggestions, seeks to help the caregiver understand Alzheimer's better and gain insight into handling specifics situations faced by all families caring for loved one with Alzheimer's disease.

By focusing not just on the patient with Alzheimer's, but also the caregivers' needs and feelings, this Caregiver's Support Kit® will try to present a realistic, yet hopeful, picture of what it means to care for someone who day by day becomes more helpless, frustrated, and dependent on your kindness and compassion.

As you embark on this journey of pain and discovery, please understand that you are not alone. There are more than 5.2 Americans with Alzheimer's today — and just as many families trying to deal with its effects on their lives. Even more important, though, there are many places and people you can turn to for help. Some of these will be discussed in the pages of this *Caregiver's Support Kit*®.

Below is a true story — one that will perhaps remind you of your own discovery about a person you love.

*****

It was a marriage that, for 25 years, had been made in heaven. Tom and his wife, Joan, had a storybook romance and a wonderful life together — filled with three beautiful children, a nice house, yearly vacations, and plenty of good friends.

One day, without warning, things began to crumble, but the reason for it only became apparent much later. Tom says it began quietly and gradually. First, he noticed that Joan spoke less and seemed more and more withdrawn. At the urging of friends and relatives, Tom took Joan to their family physician, who found nothing wrong.

But Joan remained withdrawn. She also began showing signs of anxiety, fretfulness, and irritability. Tom soon became aware that Joan wasn't taking care of the simple things she had managed for years: paying the bills, balancing the checkbook — even cleaning house and cooking. Joan had always been a neat, orderly person who prided herself on staying on top of things.

Tom suspected something was seriously wrong. He discovered bills and checks tucked away in unlikely places in the house. He found stale bits of food left in corners of the bedroom. Personal belongings and money were stashed away in the backs of drawers and cupboards, as though Joan were trying to hide them.

Tom was afraid to ask Joan about this changed behavior, thinking that most likely it was a temporary depression or perhaps the "change of life." Without saying a word, he took over the household duties and made a point of routinely returning her misplaced objects to their proper place.

But things just got worse and her forgetfulness more persistent.

Neighbors and friends began telling Tom that Joan had given them large sums of money or precious possessions, sometimes saying it was for "safekeeping," sometimes as outright gifts. They would return these to Tom, knowing full well that Joan was not acting rationally.

Thinking that a vacation might alter her mood or help her return to her former self, Tom took Joan to Europe. That's when he became aware she couldn't manage on her own. She had become almost mute and incapable of doing simple things for herself. Tom had to make all the decisions about what she ate, bought, and saw on their trip.

Finally, Tom sat Joan down in their hotel room and told her he felt she should see a doctor when they returned home. They both cried. That was the beginning of their shared journey with Alzheimer's.

*****

With this realization, Tom and Joan joined ranks of American families who have been robbed — robbed of fathers, mothers, husbands, wives, brothers, sisters, and dear friends. Robbed by a disease that destroys its patients' golden years.

The robber is called Alzheimer's disease.

And we must do everything in our power to reclaim what we can from this inhuman thief. We must work diligently to renew our relationships with our loved ones, so that we can help restore the humanity and dignity that Alzheimer's seeks to strip away.

Help for Your Loved One

Does someone you care about have any of the following symptoms? Each question below is followed by a brief illustration of the types of problem behavior and responses that may occur when the condition is caused by Alzheimer's disease.

These symptoms don't necessarily spell a diagnosis pf Alzheimer's — only a physician can make an adequate evaluation. However, if you find that, on reflection, the person displays many of the symptoms listed below, it would be a good idea to have him examined by a physician. Early detection can make an important difference in treatment and hope.

Short-term memory lapses:

1. Does your loved one forget what happened a minute ago—or not understand what's taking place right at the moment?

a. Mrs. Meyer hung up the phone after talking with her daughter about their dinner plans. She went into the living room where her husband was sitting and immediately began complaining that she wished her daughter would call, since they were supposed to make plans for dinner. Her husband asked her who she had been talking to on the phone, and she couldn't remember.

b. Ray began coming into the kitchen around dinner time and finding Marge had left a number of dishes half completed or discarded: vegetables were peeled and in a pot but the heat had been turned off, a roast left in the oven for hours was sorely overcooked, and noodles were dumped into a pan with no water. Marge had prided herself on her cooking abilities and had prepared masterful meals for her family for years. Yet, now her mind was no longer on what she was preparing. It was as though she didn't care anymore.

2. Does he seem disoriented with respect to time?

Mr. Harris would arrive at his daughter's house for dinner, take off his hat and coat and, a few minutes later, would begin insisting it was time to go home. His wife and daughter thought he was just being rude. If he didn't get his way, however, he could become frustrated and angry.

3. Do familiar objects often strike the person as unfamiliar?

Laura had bought her husband Tim a plush rocking chair as a retirement present ten years ago. Now Tim would no longer sit in it, claiming it was "someone else's chair." He repeatedly asked where his chair had gone. Laura tried buying him another chair, which he himself picked out. A few months later, he launched into the same tirade, saying this, too, was not his chair.

Memory can be difficult for any number of reasons, not all of them connected to Alzheimer's. While these memory lapses — particularly if they are frequent — may be indicative of Alzheimer's, a careful assessment by a medical professional is advised. The clinical issues involved are very complicated.

Irrational behavior/mood swings

4. Is your loved one overly anxious about routine activities like shopping, dressing, or eating?

a. Joe's eyes welled up with tears as he tried unsuccessfully to lace and tie his shoes. He couldn't

5

tell left from right, didn't understand how the laces went into the shoes, and wasn't sure what purpose it would serve him to tie them anyway. Frustrated, he kicked the shoes under the bed and locked himself in the bathroom.

b. Barbara told her mother they would stop at the post office and she would run in and get some stamps. When she got back into the car minutes later, her mother, sobbing and angry, complained that Barbara was deserting her. No amount of reassurance would calm her mother. She also could not convince her mother that she had been gone just a few moments.

5. *Does she often disguise her confusion or forgetfulness with paranoia and blame others for the problem?*

Mrs. Wright chronically mislaid her cooking utensils, scattering them in various rooms throughout the house. Every Tuesday while playing cards with her friends, she would complain to them that her husband was stealing her pots and pans and trying to drive her crazy. Her friends counseled her to confront him, thinking the problem had to do with her husband's, not their friend's, behavior.

One tragic result of the irrational, alienating behavior of the person with Alzheimer's is that she may begin to lose friends. As the wife of an Alzheimer's patient put it: "you might as well put a sign on the door that says 'leprosy' because that's exactly what's going to happen to you. You're going to be deserted." Of course, an early, proper diagnosis, shared with friends, can go a long way toward counteracting the "hands off" behavior of uncomprehending friends.

Communication breakdowns:

6. *Does your loved one exhibit problems expressing himself? Will he frequently forget the names of simple things?*

Barny often can't remember his son's name. If his wife Denise talks to him about "Jeff," Barny knows who she is talking about. But if Barny is reminiscing about his family, there are days when he is too confused to remember Jeff's name — or the names of his other children.

Patients have trouble **naming** familiar things. Even when they retain the name (e.g., sink, toothbrush), they often forget its function or purpose. Fear of confusion usually results, even when dealing with ordinary objects or activities (bathing, washing, eating).

7. *Is he often unable to complete a sentence, or does he have a tendency to run fragments of thoughts one after another in random order?*

Here's an example of rambling, incoherent speech: "I know that if I … it's a matter of time and place … you must see that he cannot be my son, my father — not without the suit coat … it's chilly where … been outside?"

It's not unusual for the Alzheimer's patients to rattle off parts of phrases he recalls from previous speech. His ability to mimic speech patterns is not impaired, and it often seems as though his thinking just gets constantly sidetracked in mid-thought. What can be difficult for people with Alzheimer's is to finish the thoughts and link them coherently with other thoughts.

8. *Has he often ignored or grossly misinterpreted written instructions you leave for him? Is he, in general, inattentive, forgetful, and excessively willful?*

a. Muriel left Fred a message on the kitchen counter: "I've gone to the doctor's. Please take the chicken out of the freezer to thaw before I cook it." Fred promptly put the chicken, wrapper and all, in the microwave, and turned it on. Then he called a cab and went to his doctor's office. When Muriel arrived home, she found that the plastic wrapper had melted into the burnt chicken.

Complicated messages are usually too much for the Alzheimer's patient to handle. He is liable to choose words or phrases that he can still recognize and provide his own meanings to them. Alzheimer's patients cannot follow **multiple** commands. ("Go to the kitchen and get me a paper towel.") You must use single, simple, and direct orders.

b. Jim and Marie were married for 44 years. When Jim started getting forgetful, he would often turn to Marie and say "Who are you? What are you doing in my house?" if she answered she was his wife and had every right to be in their house, he would get upset and threaten to call the police and have her evicted.

While none of these symptomatic behaviors is exclusively connected with Alzheimer's disease, this example comes closest to being characteristics of the course of the disease —in particular, the masking of forgetfulness with difficult, obstreperous behavior.

Loss of coordination

9. Does she have difficulty with simple movements such as walking or manual skills such as writing her name, dressing, or dialing a telephone?

Mrs. Barnes had always been energetic walker. Now, however, she had difficulty just going from room to room in her house. She often tripped over her own feet. She would raise her legs far higher than she needed to, not fully aware of spatial relations about her. Or she would drag one leg as though she was gradually forgetting how to walk.

People with Alzheimer's gradually "unlearn" the basic functions they acquired in their early life. If it's a woman, perhaps she can no longer sew, knit, or measure and cook foods. For a man, perhaps it's the inability to use a screwdriver, change a light bulb, or drive a car.

Warped or nonexistent sense of time:

10. Does he seem unable to measure the passing of time, sometimes asking repeatedly what time it is, or at other times not realizing that hours and hours have passed?

Arthur was beginning to pace up and down the hallways all night long. He would nap during the day, because he seemed unable to sleep at night. Some nights, he would wake his wife up every ten minutes and ask her the time. When she told him the time, saying "You asked me that ten minutes ago," he would vehemently deny it. He claimed, to the contrary, that it had been several hours since he was up.

She sometimes found him working with his power saw in the wee hours of the morning, sawing planks of wood into small segments. From the debris on the floor, she guessed he had been at it for hours on end.

11. Will she get confused about how to read the time off a clock and know what time it means in terms of her daily routine?

Judy waited for her daughter to come home from work and cook for dinner. Her daughter was always punctual, coming in the front door at 5:20 every evening. But when the daughter arrived home, she found her mother in angry tears, pointing at the clock and saying "Where have you been? I thought you were gone for good!" But the clock on the wall indicated 5:20.

*****

If you can answer "yes" to a substantial number of these questions, chances are you should have your loved one undergo a thorough medical examination.

This is by no means an exhaustive list of early Alzheimer's symptoms, nor are these disorders exclusive to Alzheimer's. but that is precisely why you should see a doctor or medical specialist as soon as possible, to determine what the problem may be — and, if it is Alzheimer's, to take the necessary precautions so that your loved one won't put him- or herself in grave danger.

As one doctor has put it, "If you notice that your memory is giving you problems, you probably don't have Alzheimer's. if your spouse notices that your memory is giving you problems and you don't, go see somebody."

Since Alzheimer's patients most often maintain an outward appearance of well-being, their erratic, bizarre behavior is quite often not taken as a sign of illness, but rather just oddness or "nuttiness." Because Alzheimer's symptoms can easily be mistaken for nonmedical conditions, they are often considered to be completely unrelated to disease — and mistreated as such.

Some forgetfulness and confusion occur naturally in the aging process, but if these become chronic or severe, the problem may well be the manifestations of a "hidden" illness such as Alzheimer's. Many dementias have symptoms virtually identical to Alzheimer's, but they differ in that they **do** have cures and effective treatments. It is therefore critical to obtain a thorough examination to arrive at the most definite diagnosis possible.

In addition to Alzheimer's, there are many disorders involving loss of memory and other intellectual functions, some of which can be easily treated. These dementias are also illnesses, not the natural consequence of advancing years. However, some of these **are** reversible if treated properly and in timely fashion.

Even when the diagnosis is Alzheimer's, advances in science and the wealth of resources available for improving life for Alzheimer's patients and their families have changed our outlook on this difficult disease: Today, there is hope where there was little before.

Awareness must begin at home, which is why diagnosis is so vitally important. You can never have too much information on the symptoms that are and are not part of the disease. For example, a medical condition unrelated to Alzheimer's may be exaggerating the Alzheimer's symptoms or placing the patient at risk of illness or injury; this medical condition needs to be treated separately as soon as it is identified as such. With a full, thorough diagnosis, the family can rest easier, knowing that all problems with the patient that **can** be fixed are being taken care of.

Early detection also means there is time for the family to be properly instructed in the best treatment methods. And when the family is fully informed, the behavioral problems of the Alzheimer's patient can be minimized — or at least the negative effects on the caregivers can be softened. Now, while your loved one may never display certain forms of symptomatic behavior, if you can anticipate difficulties in dealing with him, they somehow become less difficult because you knew about them in advance. This is true even as the patient moves into the later phases of the disease. In these ways, guidance by medical professionals can be life-saver for the caregivers.

Once your loved one has been diagnosed, it is critical that you also look to other sources of help. Keep an eye open for community resources at your disposal — meal and transportation services, free medical testing, volunteer visitors, and support groups. Gather as much data as you can in order to make informed decisions about living arrangements and health care. You will also want to have the latest results of research, so you know the progress of knowledge of the causes of Alzheimer's and the treatments that show most promise.

Don't hesitate to ask for outside support and guidance as your loved one progresses through the steps of this disease! Many of Alzheimer's and the treatments that show most troublesome symptoms **can be** managed — with a little help from your friends, your physicians, and your community.

Elements of Caring

The expense and caring for your loved one with Alzheimer's can be extremely costly. An d the financial drain can be made worse by lack of knowledge about the disease. Planning and foresight can make a critical difference in treatment option chosen as well as the toll that care can take on a family's resources.

The real costs of Alzheimer's aren't in the diagnosis or treatment, but in the **care** of patients. Bear in mind that many Alzheimer's patients live from six to twenty years after they are diagnosed.

At each stage of the disease, patients display particular behaviors and dysfunctions, requiring different types of treatment and care. By the time they have reached the middle to late stages of the disease, patients require unusually large amounts of care, from either family caregivers or nursing professionals.

For example, in nursing homes, professional staff have noted that they spend a disproportionate amount of their time with Alzheimer's patients, particularly those that still walk around unaided, simply because these people get themselves into hazardous situations most often. They also can forget to eat (or forget **how** to eat), so they often need to be prompted, reminded, or hand-fed. Most patients lost weight over time for a variety of medical reasons.

In recent years, a number of in- and out-patient special care units have been created specifically for patients with dementia (an umbrella term for Alzheimer's and several other closely related brain-destroying conditions). Some of the design and cost considerations that go into such a unit include:

- making sure doors and outside gates cannot be easily opened, so patients cannot wander off,

- maintaining a ratio of patients to staff that allows staff to monitor the movements of patients almost continually, to minimize injuries and serious accidents,

- placing visual clues (colors, identification tags) to help patients remember their way and maintaining a separate medication cabinet (rather than usual cart propelled through the hallways) for the safety of the patients,

- addressing the memory and communications needs of patients with sensory stimuli ("memory boards" where they clip photographs and other reminders; pets and children they can touch; baking and cooking activities),

- planning additional meals and beverage breaks to keep patients' weight normal levels and prevent dehydration,

- monitoring the feeding of patients, depending upon the stage of dementia (the potential danger of choking is quite high with Alzheimer's patients),

- providing a steady stream of structured, daily activities and group functions led by trained staff, which keep patients busy and stimulated, and

- creating programs that get other family members involved in visiting the unit and participating in group activities.

While these considerations are particularly appropriate to in-patient homes for dementia patients, they certainly apply as well to the design and layout of Alzheimer's day-care facilities — or even to modifications that must be made to the patient's house if the patient is to remain at home.

"Alzheimering" your home means protecting hot surfaces like light bulbs and radiators, talking away small objects that can go into the mouth, removing sharp objects and surfaces from the patient's reach, putting medications and toxic substances in a safe place, adapting the bathtub and toilet with grab bars to protect against slipping, covering slippery floors and securing rugs firmly to the floor, locking doors to the basement and attic stairs, keeping all house and car keys well hidden, and maintaining adequate stove safety and flame control. When keeping an Alzheimer's patient in the home, caregivers must resolve all problems connected with access, electric cords and outlets, locks (particularly to prevent wandering), the yard (especially if there's a swimming pool), and the car.

A sampling of home care equipment that will help make your home safe for the later-stage Alzheimer's patient would include plastic faucet handles that are easier for movement-impaired persons to use... security lights in the event of a power outage... time switches that turn household appliances on and off as you program them... one-way intercom to let you keep an ear on the patient in another room... "potty chairs," bedpans, and bed supports... suction plates and cups... and wheelchairs, hydraulic lifts, and stairway elevators as needed when the patient is no longer ambulatory.

The following checklist presents some basic objects caregivers can get to help the patient find his way around:

1. A medication dispenser, so **you** know, as well as the patient when pills should be taken.

2. A magnifying glass, so that small print on bottles and elsewhere can be easily read. It may even be useful in reading, watching can be easily read. It may even be useful for reading, watching television, or telling the time. (For patients who need to know the time, a watch with large hands and number can also be useful.)

3. Marketing tape, in particular colors, which you can use to mark pathways to the bathroom, kitchen, or the patient's bedroom. This will ease the strain on the patient's memory. (You will have to be very careful with this, however, because many persons with Alzheimer's cannot discriminate between a strip of tape on the floor and a step —so they may be become hesitant about moving forward. This technique is usually more successful in the early stages of the disease.)

4. An identification bracelet, in case the patient should wander from home or somehow find himself alone in a strange place. You may also want to include medical information on the bracelet — this way, a rescuer will know that the patient's confusion results from Alzheimer's.

5. Warning labels to let the patient know that opening certain drawers and touching certain surfaces are dangerous. It is best if these are in symbol form, rather than in words the patient may no longer understand.

For example, you may wish to adopt the international sign for "no," a red circle with a diagonal line drawn through it.

Of course, you will also want to offer the patient distractions that are stimulating, simple, and pleasurable. Here are some possibilities to consider:

1. Play tapes of soothing music (particularly music that is familiar to them). This should have a calming or mildly stimulating effect on the patient.

2. Give him seeds to plant and watch grow. This allows the patient to feel a sense of purpose, an ongoing responsibility that only he can take care of. One suggestion for the type of plant is a sunflower: it's easy to care for, and once the seeds have grown, you put the plant in the back yard, so the patient can watch birds feed off the plant.

3. If the patient likes animals, having a house pet around can be a good source of distraction as well. We don't suggest bringing a new pet into the house, unless you are sure it is domesticated and relatively harmless. (If you have a cat, you should consider having its claws removed.) You will need to stay alert to the fact that the patient's attitude toward the pet may suddenly change.

4. Surround the patient with familiar objects such as a favorite blanket, a shawl, or a doll. These can serve as conversation pieces; more importantly, they will reassure the patient that he is in familiar, safe surroundings.

5. Show favorite old movies — including silent pictures. These can be enjoyable for certain patients, just as the older music can help bring back recollections.

6. Encourage family members to join together in activities with the patient. Group or family activities help alleviate the loneliness the Alzheimer's patient often feels.

7. Schedule regular visits from friends or relatives. Having visitors stimulates the patient, but visits should be kept relatively brief, so the patient does not become unduly tired or frustrated.

8. In the earlier stages of the disease, patients may find help and comfort from a support group made up of others suffering from Alzheimer's.(Caregivers will definitely benefit from support groups of their peers.) Contact your state Agency on Aging for more information about support groups in your area.

9. Finally, certain "low-risk" activities, such as taking the patient for a ride in the country, can provide fruitful diversion for both the patient and the caregivers.

Even when you can't spend time with the patient, you will need to see that he is always comfortable. You may wish to order a bed or chair from a hospital supply company, adapted to the needs of patients who are immobile for long periods. Be careful to dress the patient in warm, somewhat loose clothing that is easy to wear and wash. Special items of clothing made with velcro snaps instead of buttons or zippers are particularly helpful to patients who lose manual dexterity.

Finally, but no less important, please bear in mind that you want to do whatever is in your power to let the

patient hold onto this his dignity and self-esteem.
This includes asking him to share in chores and duties, deferring to his decisions (where appropriate), listening carefully to what he has to say, and encouraging him to share his feelings and concerns.

Remember that, although Alzheimer's disease kills the person's mind, it does not kill the person inside. You must respect that person whenever possible — even though it may be harder to gain access to the unique personality beneath the ravages of the disease. You'll be glad you made the effort.

Understanding Alzheimer's Disease

What is Alzheimer's Disease?

Contrary to what many people think, Alzheimer's disease is not a normal part of aging. It is a disease in which the nerve cells in the area of the area of the brain that control memory, thinking and judgment are damaged, and the normal transmission of messages between cells is affected. Messages are passed between nerve cells by neurotransmitters. It has been found that one particular transmitter is absent in the brain of Alzheimer's sufferers. During the course of the disease, the thinking center of the brain shrinks, which in turn limits the ability of the brain to function at optimal level. The nerve cells, develop changes (detectable after death at autopsy only), called neuroticplaques and neurofibrillary tangle.

What about Diagnosis?

There is no one test available to determine whether a person has Alzheimer's disease. It is actually diagnosed by ruling out all other conditions that may cause memory loss. A positive diagnosis is made on the basis of the number and concentration of tangles in the short-term memory center of the brain.

Depression and Memory Loss

In the early stages of disease, depression may sometimes be present. The sufferer becomes distressed at what is happening — he recognizes that his memory is becoming increasingly poor. If diagnosed in an early stage of Alzheimer's disease, the "accompanying depression" usually improves with medication, even though the memory loss associated with Alzheimer's disease is still there.

Stage of Alzheimer's Disease

Although the course of the disease is unpredictable, it has been observed that the symptoms tend to fall into three stages that often overlap.

Stage 1 (Duration 2-4 Years):

Leading up to and Inclusive of Diagnosis

The primary symptoms is that short-term memory is noticeably affected. Other symptoms that may occur with varying intensity are:

- difficulty in concentrating
- poor judgement
- hesitancy about doing things that once cane easily
- sometimes problems with finding the right expression or word
- often withdrawn
- some perceptible changes may occur in personality
- anxiety about not being able to remember as well
- anxiety about what is happening to him
- difficulty coming to decisions

Why is an Evaluation Necessary?

It is very important that the medical-neurological evaluation be done to rule out whether treatable conditions are causing the symptoms. Confusion, disorientation and severe forgetfulness can arise from a variety of causes, including dehydration, malnutrition, improper use of medications, excessive alcohol use, emotional and physical traumas, acute infections and relocation. These conditions may cause a temporary delirium which is reversible once the cause is identified and treated. Alternately, the care-recipient who exhibits

21

"senility" may actually be very depressed; this condition too, can be alleviated, when a proper diagnosis is made.

There are also irreversible conditions other than Alzheimer's that may cause some of the same symptoms — for example, small strokes and cerebral arteriosclerosis. While these conditions are not treatable, their courses are different and in some cases more benign than Alzheimer's disease.

A proper medical diagnosis is the first step in dealing with the disease. The diagnosis is one of exclusion. There is presently no test available which can determine with certainty whether one has the disease. Rather a presumptive diagnosis is made, as other conditions are ruled out.

It is normal to feel hopeless and helpless when confronted with the diagnosis. You may even feel anger and the majority of caregivers go into denial, just not wanting to accept what is happening. However, information about the different stages of the disease and how to cope (much of it learned from caregivers who have already walked the path) can be very helpful.

Managing the Needs in Stage 1

Once the diagnosis is confirmed, work toward setting up a care-plan for the future and arrange the sufferer's legal and financial affairs, while he feels that he still has some control over those affairs.

Plan Ahead

A Care Plan

It is important to understand what demands the different stages may make on your time and energies.

Read everything you can find about the disease and its challenges.

Hold a family conference and talk about how the future requirements of care can be divided up among family members. Write down the decisions that are reached. Identify the services and professionals known as the "formal support system" before you need them. Learn ahead of time what their functions and limitations are, how to access them, whether any services are free, funded, or are fees based on income level. A care-plan will make all the difference in how you cope with the course of the disease.

Financial and Legal Planning

Consult a lawyer and financial advisor about what legal and financial arrangements will be needed. This will help avoid what can sometimes be difficult problems later on. As far as possible include the person with Alzheimer's disease in discussions; this may allay some of his fears.

Although he may not have many financial resources, expert advice should be sought. Many advisors will provide a first interview free of charge. Such advisors may include lawyers, insurance agents, accountants, tax consultants, bankers and bank trust officers and certified financial planners. Generally one principal advisor will work with the person with Alzheimer's and his family; where necessary, consulting with others on your behalf to plan for the Alzheimer's sufferer's total legal and financial needs.

To find a competent advisor, you may start with the family's lawyer. Or ask friends and family members whether they know of a competent professional. Or call the local Bar Association; they have an Attorney Referral

Service. Ideally the advisor should someone who is experienced in dealing with situations in which the client has Alzheimer's or a related disorder. **Before** you go for the consultation, establish whether the initial interview is free of charge and what the follow-up fees are, and for what services.

It is extremely helpful to organize documents into categories relating to the Alzheimer's sufferer's legal and financial affairs (e.g. debts, such as mortgage, car loans, credit card charges, insurance premiums, etc.) and then make a list of assets (stocks, bonds, saving accounts, property owned) before going to the actual appointment.

It probably will not be easy to talk about your family member's private affairs with him: in fact he may be very reluctant. Try to make him understand that it is in his longer-term best interests. As his condition worsens there may be added medical and living expenses; it is useful for families to know what assets are available to meet such costs. Additionally talk to all the professionals involved in any way with his legal and financial affairs, and explain what is happening. In fact you may need a lawyer to help you get access to some records.

Among the documents and certificates you should try to locate are the following (being cognizant that bank books, stock certificates, etc. may be kept in strange places — hidden away in drawers, on top of wardrobes, under the mattress, in old boxes in the attic, basement, etc.):

• wills

• bank books and statements

- stock and bond certificate sand updated statements from brokerage firms

- safety deposit boxes

- personal loans

- trust accounts

- documents re Individual Retirement Accounts

- income tax records

- pension notices

- deeds, property tax statements on any property

- evidence of any collections, i.e. antiques, art.

Learn what income and other resources can later be called upon to pay bills for care. Income may be available from a wide range of sources; for instance, Social Security, pensions, checking accounts, dividends, convertible assets, individual retirement accounts, r gifts from children or a spouse. Sources of insurance may be health insurance, Medicare, Medicaid, life insurance may VA coverage, etc. Be sure to check the clauses in any Health Insurance Policies to see whether they cover persons with Alzheimer's disease; often these policies contain an exclusion clause.

Expenses that may ultimately be incurred could be: disability aids (adaptation of the house such as ramps, rails, etc.); hired-in help to do chores or meal preparation, transportation costs, for instance, to and from adult day care or clinics; some regular nursing support (this may be essential in stage three); incontinence gear and easy-to-manage clothing.

As the condition is in its early stages, the individual may still be considered sufficiently legally competent to draw up a Will. Powers of Attorney are also useful; in some states, they may be simple or durable. A power-of-attorney is a written is a written document that allows one person to make certain decisions on behalf of another — the power give one person the legal right to manage the finances, property and/or other legal matters on behalf of another person. The person granting the power must be competent and fully understand the power-of-attorney agreement at the time it is written. A Simple Power of Attorney ends when a person becomes incompetent. A Durable Power of Attorney remains in effect even after the impaired person becomes incompetent.

Another instrument that can be very helpful is that of representative payee. A "payee" is someone who can receive and use an impaired person's benefits in the best interests of that person. At the time when the person can no longer manage his benefits, this option payees. Note that the Department of Veteran Affairs, can appoint payees. Note that the Department of Veteran Affairs calls such a person "fiduciary" ; the Social Security Administration calls them "representative payees" ; state social services, health or welfare departments sometimes use the term "protective payee." (Note too that terms differ from state to state.) When setting up a financial plan, if a considerable amount of property is involved, you should ask the advisor about trusts. Briefly, a trust instrument transfers property or money from one person to another, with certain conditions attached. The trust is managed by a third by a third person. The person creating the trust is called the "trustor" (here it will be the impaired person). The person who receives the benefit of the trust is called the "beneficiary" ; the person who manages the trust is called the "trustee." A lawyer or banker can advise what type of trust will best meet the required needs.

Ultimately, a person with Alzheimer's will lose what is called "legal competence," which is the power to manage personal, financial or legal affairs. In this case it will become necessary for someone else to make decisions on his behalf. Therefore, it is prudent to plan in advance who should be the person to make those decisions. A lawyer can advise on the options available. The most commonly used legal tools are a "guardianship" or a "conservatorship." Usually a conservatorship is the more limited form of the two, in that **a conservator manages the impaired person's fund only. A guardian on the other hand, manages both personal and financial affairs.** Note that in some cases, as stated above, another choice is a "durable power of attorney." The Alzheimer's sufferer should discuss all options with his lawyer.

Helping Your Care-Recipient Cope

Your care-recipient will be upset about what the future holds. He needs to be reassured that the family will see that he is cared for. He needs to continue to feel that he is a valued family member.

Be very vigilant about keeping him as involved as possible in the family's activities and decision-making; this will help him to cope with his own anxiety.

Don't talk about his memory loss in front of him and certainly not as though he is not there; such behavior on your part, can be very upsetting and demeaning for him.

He will generally be lucid a lot of the time during this phase. To help his confidence, make sure that he continues to keep as much to the former pattern of daily living as is possible.

Don't allow him to become withdrawn because he can't remember short-term events and conversation very well.

Don't be demanding about normal daily activities. An example is letting him dress himself even though it takes time. Be patient; not critical. You can assist him by setting his clothes out in the order of putting on.

He will almost certainly still be able to manage simple chores which do not tax his memory, so involve him; it will help him to maintain his dignity.

If he tends to get lost when he goes on errands put his name and address in his wallet to make him feel more secure.

In the event that he forgets the names of people he knows well, prompt him discreetly, to help him save face.

Don't confront him with complex, challenging decisions or questions; if you do, you will almost certainly add to his confusion.

Stage 2 (Duration 2-10 Years): *Following Diagnosis*

This stage is characteristically affected by more pronounced memory loss and even shorter memory span. Other symptoms may include:

- repeating statements
- real difficulty remembering friends' and family members' names

- restlessness, especially at night and during late afternoon (called 'sundowning')

- fear of getting into the bathtub

- real difficulty dressing

- perceptual-motor problems

- increased difficulty organizing thoughts

- problems with reading, working with numbers and writing

- more and more difficulty locating the right word

- suspiciousness, sometimes irritability

- hearing or seeing things that aren't there in fact

- perceptual-motor problems

- increased difficulty organizing thoughts

- problems with reading, working with numbers and writing

- more and more difficulty locating the right word

- suspiciousness, sometimes irritability

- hearing or seeing things that aren't there in fact

Usually at some time during this stage, there is a need for constant supervision.

Managing the Problems Associated with Stage 2

This period of the disease is very demanding on the caregiver. Generally she is required to deal with problem behaviors that are alien to her experience. The fact that it is a loved one who is involved, makes the challenge even more exhausting. Help with memory aids — e.g., a large sign on the toilet door; laying his clothes out in the right order; leaving around family photos taken sometime ago.

Watch for Triggers Which Set Off Difficult Behaviors

Coping with Restlessness and Wandering

Restlessness often occurs late in the afternoon or early evening. Researchers do not understand why. Try to identify what makes him fidgety, want to leave, or pace through the house.

Locks on gates can help to keep him from getting off the property. If he wanders get an identity bracelet for him, notify the police and neighbors in the propensity and keep a current photograph of him handy for reference.

If you follow him, do not startle him by dashing up and grabbing his arm. Try to appear unconcerned and persuade him to go back with you. You may have to walk a bit before you succeed. Note his patterns — does he tend to go off in one particular direction; does he appear confused or lost?

Coping with Repetitiveness

He will be anxious about being left alone and may follow you to feel reassured that you are close by. Constant questions or statements may be part of the behavior. This can become exhausting.

It is important to recognize that the behavior is not deliberate; he doesn't realize what he is doing.

Try to distract him with a small snack, sitting down and talking about the "old days" with a family photo album, with making that time bath-time; with music, a television or radio program or asking family or friends to call or come by at that time of day.

Coping with Fear of Bathing

It is of course important to good health to keep the person clean. Many Alzheimer's sufferers develop a fear of water and/or a fear of getting undressed and into the bath.

If it is a fear of getting down into the bath, he may be happier using a bath seat or taking a shower. If he is upset about getting undressed, then you may convince him to wrap a towel around him while he is immersed in the water. This will make washing more difficult, but it may work.

Coping with Hallucinations or Delusions

He may believe he hears, sees or smells what no-one else can. He may get up in the middle of the night to answer the door, hear bells, hear voices, see things in the room. This can be trying to deal with.

Among measures you can take is never to challenge him. Remember he is not rational and will not understand your logic. Try to avoid having any shadows in the area of the house he is in. at night, a night light may provide enough light to take away it is that triggers these hallucinations.

Coping with Hoarding

Hoarding is a behavior that can make a caregiver irritable. The person may hoard "treasures"; other people's things or even food. It is dangerous for him to hoard and then eat food as he may become ill.

Watch the pattern of his hoarding. Providing him with a special drawer or bag may satisfy this need to be busy and secretive.

Coping with Suspiciousness and Accusations

One of the behaviors that sometimes occurs is to accuse other people, even one's own family members of theft or trying to poison him. This can be upsetting and highly embarrassing. It is necessary to remind yourself that it is a symptom of the sad condition he is in.

Explain to anyone he suggests has stolen from him that he does have a disease of the brain. When people understand what is going on, their indignation generally fades.

Coping with Him Not Remembering Who You are

This can be very distressing. Perhaps you are his wife of many years, a child whom he adored, a brother or sister, yet he doesn't recognize you. Again, ty to accept that it is the disease causing the problem.

You may at this stage begin the grieving process, as you will have lost touch with the person you dearly loved—there is no longer any meaningful communication. Perhaps you will need to talk to a professional about your feelings.

Developing Better Communication Skills

Good communication skills can be helpful in every life situation; they are especially important when caring for somebody suffering from Alzheimer's disease. The following are some useful strategies:

- Speak clearly and slowly

- Do not use long sentences or ask several questions at once. (Use simple binary "yes"- no" questions.)

- Be patient; you may have to rephrase your questions.

- Remove loud noises or harsh lighting.

- Sit where he can watch your face.

- Be cognizant of your body language.

- Do not interrupt him.

- Be ready to quietly help him finish a thought.

- Do not contradict him or use an aggressive tone.

- Don't ask questions when the sufferer is showing signs of agitation.

- Help him to preserve his dignity, for instance, by ignoring the fact that he may not be able to remember from one second to the next.

- If you notice his agitation level increasing, try to divert him: music, a snack, chatter about the family, a walk in the garden, helping with some small chore — any one of these diversions may be enough to distract him and so prevent him from becoming upset because he can't follow.

You are principally concerned with the present; he, on the other hand, thinks about the past; sometimes, his mind goes right back to his early childhood. Of course you will become bored by hearing the same story over and over, but try to ask questions to make him feel that he is at least being listened to: it will help. If he drifts off in the middle of a thought, gently try to bring him back on course or introduce an activity so he will forget what he was talking about. Having mementos of his previous job, e.g. a picture of his farm, if he was a farmer; a picture of the car he rebuilt, if he was a mechanic, can help to stimulate long-term memories.

Implementing Earlier Decisions about Managing His Finances

You may have gotten a clear picture of the financial situation during stage 1, and you may have even set up the machinery to deal with the problems as they eventuated. Now it may be necessary to implement those plans, e.g. having Social Security and pension checks directly deposited into bank accounts.

What about You?

Get as much support and time off as you can possibly arrange. Use whatever respite services are available and affordable. It is vitally necessary for you to get away regularly and for longer periods of time.

Stage 3: The Terminal Phase

Symptoms typical of this stage:

- doesn't recognize himself
- unable to take care of himself
- difficulty swallowing
- sleeps longer and more fitfully
- bizarre or disturbing behaviors such as constant crying, hitting, biting, screaming, grunting noises.
- Loss of control over bladder and or bowels
- Abusive, angry, aggressive, demanding behaviors
- Bizarre sexual behaviors

Managing Stage 3

Special Care Situations
Incontinence
People with Alzheimer's disease, may become unable to control bladder and/or bowel movements — this is called becoming incontinent. The condition can be

34

distressing not only not only for the care-recipient, but for the caregiver. In fact, it is often the most distressing facet of the disease.

Coping with Angry, Aggressive Behaviors.
(Note: these behaviors do not always occur.)

- Remove photos of the person as they may confuse him even more and distress him.

- Remove mirrors as he may be startled by the image, believing it to be someone else.

- Keep all potentially dangerous implements locked away. Ensure that machinery such as lawn mowers, cars, etc. are not accessible.

- Keep emergency telephone numbers handy and those of available neighbors whose help you may need if he shows signs of attacking you.

- If he is aggressive, try not to react angrily. He does not know what he is doing.

Coping with Bizarre Sexual Behaviors
(Note: these do not occur in all cases.)

Tell yourself he doesn't know what he is doing. Try every diversionary tactic you have developed. The doctor may suggest medications.

Implementing the Final Stage of the "Care-Plan"
Generally this is a very stressful period, the care-recipient is in the terminal stage; the caregiver feels quite helpless and often times afraid of her own safety. It is vitally important to involve professionals at this stage. They can advise and guide his care; implementing the services they consider to be appropriate.

The visiting nurse will advise on home-nursing strategies, how to cope with incontinence, how to deal with weird sexual behaviors, and difficult and aggressive behaviors.

What about You?

Get respite. Share the care as much as you can with other family members. Bring in a nurse to help bathe and care for him. Try to keep in contact with other people.

Join a caregiver's support group. **You must try to take care of yourself.**

At this stage, you may become completely overwhelmed and come to the realization that you just cannot cope any longer. Nursing-home care may be the only realistic alternative.

Such a decision is never easy. It can cause you to feel inadequate, guilty and as though you are abandoning your loved one. But the care demands may just be too great.

Caring for a loved one with Alzheimer's disease can be exhausting, overwhelming, and distressing. If you plan ahead and get in help, it can be made less stressful. You will need all the patience and love you have.

"The best and most

beautiful things in the world

cannot be seen

or even touched.

They must be felt with the
heart."

Helen keller

Wandering

What is Wandering?

Wandering is a common and potentially life-threatening behavior that may accompany Alzheimer's disease. Individuals with this disease may become disoriented and lost, in their own neighborhoods or far from home. Nearly 60 percent of five million Americans with Alzheimer's disease may wander off and get lost sometime during the course of the disease, and many do so repeatedly. All patients who are ambulatory are at risk.

There are many reasons why an Alzheimer's patient wanders or walks away from home or a well-known path or area. As a first step, try to determine the reasons behind wandering by asking these questions:

Medication

Some medications have side effects that result in confusion and restlessness. Is the patient on such medications? If so, consult your physician.

Stress

Is the person trying to handle stress, noise, unpleasant people, crowding, or isolation? If so, consider changing the situation.

Time Confusion

Does the person become confused at certain parts of the day, such as the middle of the night or early evening? Does the person claim that people have been gone for days or weeks and then searches for them?

Basic Needs

Is the person looking for something specific such as food, drink, the bathroom, or companionship?

Restlessness

Does the person in a new or changed physical environment that makes him what to search for familiar objects, surroundings, or people?

Lack of Recognition

Is the person in a new or changed physical environment that makes him want to search for familiar objects, surroundings, or people?

Fear

Is the person trying to escape from something frightening? Is the person experiencing a delusion or hallucination, or has the person simply misinterpreted sights and sounds?

Past Behavior

Is the person trying to meet former obligations involving a former job, home, friend, or family member?

Other factors that may contribute to wandering include medical conditions such as stroke, or other issues such as consumption of alcohol, changes in the weather, or feeling abandoned, useless, or helpless. Wandering may be frustrating and irritating for caregivers, but it becomes a problem only when the person moves into an unsafe or unhealthy area or climate, puts others at risk, or invades others' property.

For this reason, many people who care for Alzheimer's patients decide to overlook wandering behavior until it becomes dangerous to the patient and to others. Or they permit the person to wander within safe boundaries pr follow the individual on special outings.

Action Steps

Be prepared

Be aware that wandering may or may not happen. There's no way to predict who will wander or when and how it might happen. Some people never get lost, and others get lost frequently. The best advice is to be prepared. If the person has a daily exercise routine and hasn't yet wandered, you needn't be overly concerned. However, once the person begins to wander or get lost, you should watch him more closely.

Encourage movement and exercise

Allow the person to move within the safe areas or make a shared exercise such as walking part of your daily routine. Although walking a circle might seem unusual, keep in mind that physical activity — from walking and sweeping, to rolling yarn or folding clothes — is a positive experience for the person with Alzheimer's.

Be objective

Don't take the person's wandering behavior personally. The individuals is probably trying to make sense of a world that no longer seems predictable.

Be aware of hazards

Remember that places that look safe might be dangerous for the person with Alzheimer's. For this reason, you should review the environment around your home for possible hazards, such as fences and gates, bodies of water, swimming pools, dense foliage, tunnels, bus stops, steep stairways, high balconies, and roadways where traffic tends to be heavy.

Secure your living area

Do whatever you can to keep your home safe and secure. Place locks out of the normal line of vision — either very high or very low on doors. In addition, use a double-bolt door lock, keeping the key handy for emergencies. Also use a childproof door knob that prevents the person with Alzheimer's from opening the door. Other effective safety actions include the following:

- Put hedges or fences around your patio or yard.

- Place locks on gates.

- Consider electronic buzzers, infrared electronic eye alarms, or chimes on your doors.

- Place a pressure-sensitive mat at the door or person's bedside.

- Camouflage some doors with a screen or curtain, or put a two-foot square of a dark color in front of the door knob.

- Use a recliner or rocking chair; the person may need assistance to get up.

- Use nightlights, signs, and familiar objects to help the person move around in a safe area.

- Put gates a dangerous stairwells.

Communicate with the person

Remind that you know how to find him and that you know how to find him and that he's in the right place. If possible, take the person for rides in cars or buses in addition to providing regular activity and exercise. And continually reassure the person, who may feel lost or abandoned.

Identify the patient

Investigate the Alzheimer's Association's Safe return program. You may want to invest in a discrete identification bracelet or locket that includes the person's name, telephone number, memory problem, and medical condition. Some experts have even recommended putting identification on the person's dentures or attaching a sensor to the patient's ankle or wrist. In addition, choose bright-colored marker, or reflective material. Also place identification on the person's shoes, eyeglasses, and keys.

Involve your neighbors

Inform your neighbors pf the person's condition and keep a list of their names and telephone numbers only. Although neighbors can be helpful in guiding the person home, you'll probably want to teach them how to approach the person with Alzheimer's disease by using these steps:

- Approach the person from the front.

- Introduce yourself and call or ask a name.

- Gently look for or ask to see identification.

- Offer help and reestablish the day, date and time.

- Avoid pulling or pushing the person.

- Report the patient found.

Involve the police

Some police departments keep a photo and fingerprints of people with Alzheimer's on file. Manu local Alzheimer's Association chapters sponsor some kind of identification program to help with wandering patients. If a person with Alzheimer's becomes lost, take a photo and an article of unwashed, worn clothing in a plastic bag to the police. Also have data on the following items:

- Age
- Hair color
- Blood type
- Eye color
- Identifying marks
- Medical condition
- Medication
- Dental work
- Jewelry
- Allergies
- Complexion

Offer suggestions about where the police might find the patient, such as old neighborhoods, former workplaces, or favorite places.

Be prepared for other modes of wandering

Although most wandering takes place by foot, some individuals with Alzheimer's disease have been known to drive 300 miles — sometimes in an automobile that belongs to someone else. You can prevent these problems by keeping car keys out of sight or by temporarily disabling the car by removing its distributor cap.

Resources

For additional help, the Alzheimer's Association has a nationwide program, Safe Return, to help locate and return missing people with Alzheimer's disease and other memory impairments.

Safe Return program includes:

- identification products, including wallet cards, jewelry, and clothing tags

- 24-hour, toll-free emergency crisis line

- Alzheimer's Association local chapter support

- wandering behavior education and training for caregivers and families

How does Safe Return work?

To register, a person with dementia or their caregiver fills out a simple form, supplies a photograph, and chooses the type of identification product that the registrant will wear and/or carry. This information is then entered into a national database.

If that individual wanders and is found, the person who finds him/her can call the Safe Return toll-free number located on the wanderer's identification wallet card, jewelry, or clothing tag. The Safe Return telephone operator immediately alerts the family members or caregivers listed in the database, so they can be reunited with their loved one.

If a person is reported missing by a family member or caregiver, Safe Return immediately alerts local law enforcement agencies to aid in the search. Local Alzheimer's Association chapters provide family support and assistance, while police conduct the search and rescue.

If a person is reported missing by a family member or caregiver, Safe Return immediately alerts local law enforcement agencies to aid in the search. Local Alzheimer's Association chapters provide family support and assistance, while police conduct the search and rescue.

For further information on Safe Return, call your local Alzheimer's Association chapter. For the chapter nearest you call 1-800-272-3900.

Special thanks to the Alzheimer's Association for their contribution to this chapter on wandering.

"Who will tell whether one

happy moment of love or

the joy of breathing

or walking on a bright
morning

and smelling the fresh air,

is not worth all the suffering

and effort which life implies."

Erich Fromm

Stage of Alzheimer's Disease

Although the course of the disease is unpredictable, it has been observed that the symptoms tend to fall into three stages that often overlap.

Stage	Duration	Common Symptoms
1	2-4 Years	• short-term memory loss
		• difficulty in concentrating
		• poor judgement
		• hesitancy about doing things that once came easily
		• sometimes problems with finding the right expression or word
		• often withdrawn
		• some perceptible changes may occur in personality
		• anxiety about what is happening to him
		• difficulty coming to decisions
2	2-10 Years Following Diagnostics	• repeating statements
		• real difficulty remembering friends' and family member' names
		• restlessness, especially at night and late afternoon (called 'sundowning')

47

• fear of getting into the bathtub

• real difficulty dressing

• perceptual-motor problems

• increased difficulty organizing thoughts

• problems with reading, working with numbers and writing

• more and more difficulty locating the right word

• suspiciousness, sometimes irritability

• hearing or seeing things that aren't there in fact

3   Terminal
     Phase

• doesn't recognize himself

• unable to take care of himself

• difficulty swallowing

• sleeps longer and more fitfully

• bizarre or disturbing behaviors such as constant crying-, hitting, biting, screaming, gnmting noises

• loss of control over bladder and or bowels

- abusive, angry, aggressive, demanding behaviors

- bizarre sexual behaviors

Alzheimer's Disease Centers

You may contact 27 Alzheimer's Disease Centers funded by the National Institute on Aging. Researchers at these centers are working to improve care and diagnosis for Alzheimer's patients. Many of the centers also have clinics that provide services for people with Alzheimer's.

Alabama

University of Alabama at Birmingham	205-934-3847

California

University of California, Los Angeles	3 10-794-6039
University of California, San Diego	858-622-5800
University of Southern California	213-740-7777

Georgia

Emory University/Wesley Wood Center	404-728-4888

Illinois

Indiana University	317-278-5500

Kansas

University of Kansas	913-588-0555

Kentucky

University of Kentucky	859-323-6040

Maryland

The Johns Hopkins Medical Institutions	410-955-6158

Massachusetts

Massachusetts General Hospital	617-726-1728

Michigan

University of Michigan – Clinic	734-764-6831
Research Center	734-764-2191

Minnesota

Mayo Clinic	507-284-1324

Missouri

Washington University	314-286-2881

New York

Columbia University	212-305-3300
Mt. Sinai School of Medicine/	
Bronx VA Medical Center	212-241-8329
New York University Medical Center	212-263-8088
University of Rochester	585-275-2581

North Carolina

Duke University	866-444-2372

Ohio

Case Western Reserve University	216-844-7360

Oregon

Oregon Health Sciences University	503-494-6976

Pennsylvania

University of Pennsylvania	215-662-2700
University of Pittsburgh	412-629-2700

Texas

Baylor College of Medicine	713-798-7416
University of Texas, Southwestern	214-648-9376
Medical Center	

Washington

University of Washington   206-598-7792

Communication:
The Difficult, Two-Way Street

So much depends on understanding. If caregivers misinterpret signals from the patient and act on those misinterpretations, it can result in excessive frustration for all concerned. For example: a patient asks the same question over and over again. The patient's family might think the patient "isn't trying" to understand — he wants to annoy them, he's lazy, or he could control his behavior if he wanted to. The simple truth is that the patient cannot help himself. Most often, the family gets upset and reacts harshly to the patient, but this only increases the frustrations felt by family and patient alike. It also resolves nothing.

If families are led to understand that loss of memory and other mental functions —symptoms of the disease — are at the root of Alzheimer's disease, they can also be shown that empathy is the key to supportive behavior. In other words, you don't try to reason with them ("You just asked that question and got an answer."). You calm them by being soothing or openly sympathizing with their problems ("You calm them by being soothing or openly sympathizing with their problems ("It's not important — don't worry about it.").

Of course, you must bear in mind that Alzheimer's patient's often use words in inappropriate ways. An example of the mildest form of this would be the wife who tells her husband she is "worried about a bank account," even though it was one they closed out years earlier. He may misinterpret that as a criticism of his money management and responds angrily — which only escalates her fear and insecurity. The more appropriate response for him is to reassure her that they have sufficient money to live. She is not questioning his competence or any specific details of the bank account; she is merely expressing her fear that they might not have enough money.

Caregivers must be taught specific problem-solving skills in order to deal with dilemmas brought on by these unpredictable behaviors. Here are just a few suggestions for dealing with problems of communication at each stage of the patient's disease. (There are a number of ways of defining the "stages" of Alzheimer's disease; the descriptions below are not necessarily the best in all case.)

Early to Early-Middle Stage

The patient may hesitate or delay response in the course of a conversation. He is struggling to find a word or phrase, but you must give him the time he needs to find it. Help him if he seems frustrated. Do it gently and reassuringly.

The patient may talk in circumlocutions — instead of asking for the butter, he may say "Can I have that stuff you spread on bread?" Since this will be a long-term coping mechanism in the progress of the disease, he should be encouraged to use circumlocutions, rather than being, "corrected" with the specific word.

The patient's conversation will be punctuated with digressions, brief and mild at first. Usually at this stage, the patient will bring the conversation around himself to the topic at hand; if not, a gentle reminder is appropriate.

Finally, the patient will very often correct his own communications slips in the early stage. He will try to mask his embarrassment or distress by joking about it, glossing over it, or correcting the mistake quickly and going on. Never challenge him when he tries to hide mistakes!

It is very important in communicating with Alzheimer's patients to maintain eye contact with them throughout the conversation, to speak slowly and simply (without resorting to baby talk!) to try different ways of saying the same thing when comprehension seems particularly difficult, and to respond with warmth and empathy to the patient's expressed feelings.

Middle Stage

The patient's store of factual knowledge is severely reduced. His ability to perform complex daily tasks (shopping, reading, driving) is drastically impaired.

Linguistically, this translates, first, into what is called semantic paraphasia, or the substitution of a closely related word for the forgotten word. You should work hard to interpret these misnomers within the context of the conversation and your surroundings — these will frequently yield the clues which the patient cannot give you. If you still cannot understand the sense, ask simple, direct questions of the patient, such as offering choices, listing possible words, asking the patient to describe the object or to use gestures to express his meaning.

Patients at this stage also cover up their lack of understanding by using cliches. A patient may say he has "never felt-better" to a question about his health, which may not reflect his actual condition at all. It is pointless to make the patient aware of the deception or hypocrisy, but you must guard against being taken in. Ask more questions, or be more specific about your concerns.

Digressions become more frequent, and the patient is no longer able to regain the thread of a conversation by himself. Gently, politely guide him back into the mainstream, in such a way that you do not compromise his self-respect.

The patient has begun to experience motor and coordination problems and will probably withdraw socially more and more. He will not initiate conversation very often. These difficulties can be softened by helping the patient remember his skills and abilities through the use of props and mementos. At this stage, the best questions are those that evoke reminiscences, solicit opinions, or inspire happy memories. Through these gambits, you stand the best chance of "breaking into" the shell that seems to be developing around the patient.

The patient will show severe difficulty in understanding simple phrases such as "how are you today?" and may ask you to repeat them several times. Be patient, speak slowly, and enunciate words broadly. Use expressive gestures where possible.

You must also make no connections unspoken when you speak to the patient. For example, when you tell him you are going to the store, give him simple, concrete details of what you are going to buy, how long you will be gone, and who will be in the house while you're away.

Likewise, when you instruct the patient to do something, you must be concrete and methodical. Since the patient can now follow only one direction at a time, break tasks and daily routines down into discrete, short steps. An example would be dressing in the morning, which should involve at least six or seven steps. Each piece of clothing needs to become its own task, so that the clothing is put on in the correct order.

At this stage of the patient's illness, when you speak to him you will need to address him by name, avoid all abstractions, communicate simply and in single thoughts, never change the subject abruptly, try to use a basic and over again, provide encouragement and praise, and reinforce your messages or directions as often as possible by writing them down.

Late-Middle Stage

When the illness has progressed to this stage, few of the patient's communication skills are intact. He is able to understand and speak only on the most basic levels. He will need help bathing, dressing, and eating, and he will have great difficulty expressing even the most basic needs. The patient will use general, not precise, words. For example, he might say "food" whenever he wants a particular kind of food, and you must play an elimination game with him to determine exactly what kind of food he wants.

The patient has now lost most of his expressive vocabulary and cannot talk about his thoughts and feelings other than in crude, partial terms. By singing familiar children's songs with him, you may help jog his memory for certain words. At the same time, you help him exercise his vocal cords and swallowing muscles.

Even simple words like "cup," "sink," or "comb" are no longer recognized. You will often have to resort to describing these objects and their functions in order to make yourself understood — e.g., a cup is "the round thing you hold in your hand and juice goes into it and you drink from it."

The patient might withdraw from conversation completely or chatter interminably in this stage of Alzheimer's disease. For either extreme, you may need to ask frequent questions to get him back on track and into a two-way conversation with you.

Some patients at this stage babble the same words or sounds over and over again. It may be impossible to get them to stop. They will lapse in and out of this habit. If it gets too annoying, simply leave the room for awhile and return when the patient has quieted down.

Although the temptation may be great to talk about the patient while he is present, avoid it! We don't know how much a patient at this stage still comprehends, but it is critical not to run the risk of demeaning or otherwise stripping the patient of his dignity.

You must be crystal-clear, simple and direct in your speaking with the patient. Announce your intentions, stick to tried-and-true meaningful words, and pay close attention to his silent language (facial expressions, gestures, body postures, movements) for clues as to what he may want or need.

Late Stage

The patient is now very disoriented in space and time. He probably no longer recognizes family members or close friends. Your most important communicating method at this stage is touch. It reassures, comforts, and communicates affection.

With incontinence and disturbed sleep patterns added to his previous inability's, the patient is now incapable of doing anything without assistance. And his communication is now minimal — he will babble, talk nonsense, or repeat back what you say to them (echolalia). Even hi "yes" and no "" responses to your questions are unreliable and should be tested. If you ask the patient whether he wants to eat, he may say "no" only because he can no longer connect the feeling of hunger with the idea of eating. In some cases, a one- or two-word message written down can help the patient recall that he wants "food" or needs tot go to the "bathroom." This technique can be particularly effective in dealing with the patient's basic needs.

Foreign-born patients who learned another language in their early years will frequently revert back to that tongue in this stage. If you know the basic words in that language, you may gain a distinct advantage in communicating with your late stage relative.

Gradually, at the point where you will most likely be calling on hospice care, all of the patient's cognitive functions break down: You cannot make yourself understood at all, and he can no longer express anything meaningful to you. Gesture and mime will be your last, most precious resource. Do a pantomime of what you want the patient to do — and you'll find the results surprisingly good!

These may sound like simple prescriptions, but they are extremely difficult to put into practice. The emotional wear-and-tear to the caregiver may make these "practical" measures seem callous or superfluous, but they are quite literally the only means left of communicating with the patient.

Caregivers must learn to constantly shift their expectations, to scale them back as the disease progresses, and never to forget that the patient is not deliberately being stubborn or mean.

These key strategies will make it possible to sustain a fruitful, meaningful relationship with your loved one throughout the course of the disease.

"When we truly care for ourselves, it becomes possible to care far more profoundly about other people. The more alert and sensitive to our own needs, the more loving and generous we can be toward others."

Eda LaShan

Rights of Alzheimer's Patients

Because there are so many legal and ethical questions bound up with having Alzheimer's disease, it's important to draw the lines with rights and responsibilities as carefully as possible. In the interest of compassion, it is also desirable to be as clear as possible about each person's responsibilities at each stage of the disease.

Here's a partial list of the patient's rights and what they mean to his dignity and well-being.

The Right to Know

A "conspiracy of silence" has been found to be detrimental for all serious disease — Alzheimer's is no exception. Generally, patients in the early stages know something is wrong, when they ask, they deserve to be told precisely what it is. This can help allay their fears and uncertainties.

When the patient knows what is happening to him, he can exercise informed choice about the care he will receive. While still capable of making decisions (in the earliest stages of the illness), he should be given control over what is being done with his body, and he should be granted a right to his own privacy. If he is conscious or aware of the fundamental choices to be made regarding terminal care and life-support systems, he should be consulted. Informed consent is the key element to giving the patient as much dignity and individuality as he can handle.

The Right to Grieve

Give the patient every opportunity to share his feelings and sadness with his family, friends and other caregivers. Patients can benefit from an outpouring of love and care — and assurance of constancy — from the family. Patients and family have the right to say "goodbye."

The Right to Quality Care

The patient deserves the very best in care, whether at home or in a nursing facility. Not only should the environment be free of hazards (physical dangers, possibility of wandering off), it should also be conducive to the patient's emotional well-being. Whenever possible, the patient should not be excessively constrained by medications such as tranquilizers or restrained physically for any length of time — at least, not as an alternative to well-designed, proper long-term care. The patient has a right to stimulation, whether through personal attention or programmed activities.

In the early stage of Alzheimer's, the patient can help make the decision as to the best nursing home. If he accompanies the family as they visit potential homes and has input in the decision to put him in a home.

The Right to Manage Assets

Early on, the patient and family should plan financial affairs carefully, to allow for the inevitable admission of the patient to a long-term care facility and to ensure that payment for this care won't impoverish the spouse and dependent children. You should talk to a financial advisor at the onset of symptoms. Also, have papers drawn up to designate power-of-attorney to the responsible caregiver. Prior planning in matters such as these is essential to peace of mind in the years ahead. In this way, your loved one can also be part of the decision-making process.

The Right to Consider All Health Care Options

Since an Alzheimer's patient may eventually be put on life-support machines, the patient should make decisions early on regarding the prolongation of life. Creating a living will or granting a power-of-attorney will facilitate actions the family has to take down the road — based on decisions the patient has already made. Of course, regulations regarding the prolongation and/or termination of life vary widely according to the geographic jurisdiction you fall under. You should find out about the regulations in effect in your area, so you understand the latitude you and your family have with regard to these decisions.

The Right to Participate in Research Projects

Often, participation in Alzheimer's research projects can give patients an added sense of purpose or meaning to their suffering and pain. Patients must give their consent to be subjects at an early stage, again in the form of a power of attorney or an appointed representative. In many cases, the family will be required to sign a release. Often, discussion with the patient and family is initiated in the early stage of Alzheimer's; the decision itself is dictated by the timing of the research proposal.

Just as the patients have certain rights, so the families must also bear certain responsibilities. Carrying these out not only serves the loved one who has Alzheimer's, but also helps to set limits and preserve the lives of the individual members of the family. Where possible, families should try to confront the disease with the patient and share in the grieving. They must be courageous and honest with the patient. Families must also safeguard their own self-interests, maintaining the proper balance between the demands of their own lives and those of their loved one.

The Right to Manage Assets

Early on, the patient and family should plan financial affairs carefully, to allow for the inevitable admission of the patient a long-term care facility **and** to ensure that payment for this care won't impoverish the spouse and dependent children. You

The role of professional caregivers is essential to the protection and maintenance of these rights and responsibilities. In order that both the patients and the family feel they can act courageously and decisively, they must be fully aware of the support and infrastructure provided by professional caregivers. Likewise, professionals who understand the range of problems connected with the disease can help families come to appropriate decisions and resolve emotional conflicts.

"A BEND IN THE
ROAD IS NOT
THE END OF THE ROAD.
......UNLESS
YOU FAIL TO MAKE
THE TURN."

Anonymous

Rights of Alzheimer's Caregivers

However you handle the person under your care, whatever decisions you make, you should bear in mind that you, too, have certain rights as caregiver.

The Right to Get Frustrated

If your loved one is sorely trying your patience, simply stop what you are doing, take a deep breath, and do something else.

The Right to be Occasionally Impatient

Of course, it is pointless to show your impatience to the patient, since he either will not understand or may feel hurt your impatience. Try to channel the feeling into more positive activity — talk it out with someone neutral, do something physical like housework, or take a walk.

The Right to Want Time to be Alone

Your judgement will take you only so far. The patient's constantly changing behavior will present challenges, some of which you will be unprepared to cope with adequately the first time around. You'll learn through trial and error at each stage of the disease.

The Right to Ask for Help

You have limits, which you must respect for your own sake, as well as for the patient's. Don't hesitate to call on family, friends, and community resources for help. Your doctors are clergy can make referrals.

The Right to Greive

It is not unusual for you to feel intense sadness even while your loved one is alive, because so often he doesn't seem to be the same person anymore.

The Right to Love, Lough, and be Touched

You'll still make real contact with your loved one, sometimes unexpectedly. Be open to these special moments. There are still many riches in your loved one!

The Right to Hope

Never give up. While Alzheimer's follows an inexorable course, there are moments of lucidity, slight upturns that bring relief to patient and caregiver alike. Learn to look for and gather strength from these moments.

Whatever you do, don't despair. A cure for this difficult condition will eventually be found. Perhaps during the lifetime of your loved one effective treatment will become available. Keep in touch with your sources of information, such as the National Caregiving Foundation, to find out about the latest resources and help for caregivers and patients. Death is as inevitable as birth. Care and compassion make us human.

In the meantime, know that there are many people out there who care about you and want to help you and your loved one.

The Right to Have Fun

Like a tree without the sun for nourishment, without fun in your life you are going to wither away. It is as important to have fun and recreate as it is to do work and chores. Don't discount it and don't feel guilty if you enjoy yourself from time to time. You are a person too and need to experience the same pleasures as you wish for your care receipt. Make some arrangements to go out to a movie or dinner or for a walk in the park. It's okay to have some fun.

Creating
Advocate — Not Adversaries

by Linda Morrison Combs, Ed.D.

All of us who go through the daily trials and tribulations of caregiving know that we must continually find ways to create advocates or helpers — both for our loved one as well as for ourselves. Often the family physician can be one of those sources.

I have been coping with Alzheimer's disease for almost half a century. First, as a child, with my maternal grandmother, and presently with my mother who is currently suffering with the disease. My personal experiences when seeking a diagnosis for my mother reiterated to me the need for a primary care physician who would indeed be an advocate—both for the patient, for family members, and for the caregiver.

What to look for in physician

- concerned, caring attitude that demonstrates to the patient and family member that the physician will indeed be an advocate — any demonstration of the attitude that "We are in this together. I don't have all the answers, but we'll work through this together step by step."

- Someone who offers careful, systematic testing and a simple, direct explanation of the plan for diagnosis—what test will be given, what information is needed, history, current status, drugs currently taken, diet, mood of the patient. Discussion of what will be done in terms of mental tests — simple paper/pencil tests, etc. Explanation of whether simple reflex tests will be done, CAT, EEG, or lab tests, etc.

- Preparation of the caregiver and patient prior to time of testing concerning the length of time the tests will take, how many office visits will be required, and over what period of time, etc.

- Discussion ahead of time about how the "result session" will be conducted — in person — with caregiver and patient — not over the phone, etc.

- Someone who is eager to share information about where to go for additional help — at the least, toll-free numbers should be given for places to go for assistance, depending on the condition diagnosed.

The most positive things physicians can do to assist caregivers

- See the patient at the appointed time. A doctor's waiting room can be a fearful place — especially for a demented patient.it can be very trying for caregivers who must answer the patient's question every five minutes — "When are we going home?" or "What am I doing here anyway?"

- Assume the responsibility to encourage caregivers and family members to seek emotional support — referrals to support groups, toll-free telephone number, Internet addresses, etc. Physicians should not assume that they are only responsible for the scientific diagnosis and treatment of the patient. They have a larger obligation — to act as partner and advocate for the patient and the caregiver.

- Talk about safety with the patient and caregiver — driving, falling, being careful with appliances, etc.

Make certain that the caregiver is aware that the safety of the patient is a priority.

- Talk about various other needs of the patient — diet, rest, personal care, medications, changes to watch out for in appetite, bladder and bowel functions, sitter and visiting nurses, meals on wheels, or other community services. Many of these personalized needs will depend on what the physician observes or is told by the caregiver.

- Realize that the patient you see for 20 minutes may be "superficially normal" for that period of time. If memory problems are presented, listen carefully to see if the patient is evading direct questions, covering speak for the patient.

- Multiply what you see in that 20-minute office visit by 72. (That's how many 20-minutes segments the caregiver is spending with the patient each and every day.)

- Look at the total patient — not just the charts. Look at the total person within their family structure as well. Do they currently live alone?

Do they have family support close by — or are they being cared for at a distance.

- Be genuine and empathetic — if the diagnosis is positive, words like, "Unfortunately, things will get worse, but we can work through this together," can really mean a lot to a family member, caregiver, or patient.

Some things physicians sometimes do that make caregivers and family members feel uncomfortable or dissatisfied

- Saying "nothing can be done" is irritating and simply not correct. Maybe nothing can be done about the diagnosis or about the disease — but there are lots of things that can be done to help caregivers, family members, and patients cope with a diagnosis and with any disease and its symptoms.

- If memory loss is part of the reason for seeking a diagnosis, telling caregivers or patients that progressive forgetting is a part of "normal aging" is not comforting — neither is it true.

- Talking only to the caregiver or family member — when the patient is also present — is rude and insensitive.

What patients, family members, and caregivers can do to help physicians

- In preparation for a visit to the doctor, collect medications in a bag and carry them to the appointment — all of the prescription medications as well as over-the-counter medications.

- Family members, caregiver, and patient (if still able) should talk about family history or diseases in preparation to an initial visit to a doctor. What was the cause of death of parents, grandparents, etc. compare notes of what is causing the patient to need to seek medical attention at this time — is it sudden decline, progressive decline—and in what areas. The person accompanying the patient to the doctor should take careful notes and be prepared to talk honestly and openly with the physician, reporting these conversations and observations.

- Know which doctor you are going to—and why—a specialist, a family physician, a primary caregiver, etc.

- If the patient is seeing a family doctor, a primary care physician, realizes that they are generalists and are looking for many different illnesses. If you are primarily concerned with dementia, the caregiver should be prepared to ask for a referral to a neurologist or psychiatrist.

- Engage in an open, forthright dialogue with the doctor and other health care professionals.

- Accept the reality of the diagnosis and the disease.

- Accept the limitations of the patient.

- Assume the role caregiver, spokesperson, and interpreter between the patient and doctor when it is necessary — but only when the patient is incapable.

- Do not ask or expect the physician to make decisions you as a caregiver or family member should make yourself.

- Do not expect and demand quick, easy answers. There may be no quick, easy or simple answers. Remember, you are trying to locate an advocate — not an adversary — for the caregiver and the patient.

As caregivers we must always remember that we cannot possibly supply all the care that our loved one ultimately needs. We must continually pursue help from other volunteers, organizations, professionals, and family members. The individuals and organizations we select to be a part of this vital support team can make our caregiving experiences some of the most rewarding experiences of our lifetime.

Dr. Combs is the former Assistant Secretary for Management at the Unites States Department of the Treasury. She resigned that position to become a caregiver. She is currently a speaker and author of A Long Good-Bye, Reflections on Dealing with Alzheimer's. For more information, contact: Dr. Linda Combs, 421 Cedar Trail, Winston-Salem, NC 27104. Telephone 336-748-9052, Toll Free 800-932-6627 or fax 336-723-1661.

Reminiscing

One of the most distressing early impacts of Alzheimer's or related disease on the sufferer and the family, is the person's inability to recall recent events. Long-term memory is often astoundingly intact.

Therefore, in an effort to make life more pleasurable for all concerned, it is wise to prepare a record of some information about a loved one's earlier life. This record can be written, or audio/video taped if not too disconcerting to your care-recipient. It can then be used later on to help the patient and the family have more meaningful communication.

Recent studies, funded in part by the National Caregiving Foundation, show reminiscent videos to be an additional tool used for Alzheimer's patients by their caregivers. The images are pictures selected by the caregiver with captions that are most meaningful to the patient. The background music can also be selected.

What you are trying to establish is a profile of the person's life history; so start with questions which will enable him to talk about that very early period of his life.

(The following guidance of course will need adaptation if it is a female relative.)

Early Childhood
Your Parents

- Were they born here or did they immigrate here?

- If they came as immigrants, how old were they at the time and from which country did they come?

- Was life hard for them in the early days?

- How did your father make a living?
- Were they kind?
- Who was the greatest influence on your life?

The Family
- How many brothers and sisters did you have?
- Who was your favorite brother/sister?
- Where did you live?
- Did your father change jobs often?
- Did the family have other relatives close by?
- Did the family go to church?
- Did the family have any pets?
- Did you have your own pet?
- What was he like?
- Was anyone in the immediate family ever seriously ill?
- Did you think of yourselves as poor, struggling, comfortably well off?
- Did your parents worry about money?
- Did your grandparents live with you?

School
- Who was your first teacher?
- How old were you when you went to school?
- How did you get to school?
- What was the name of your best friend; what was he like?

- Did you like school?
- Did you do well in school?
- Did you have any unfulfilled goals; e.g. becoming a doctor or farmer?
- What is your earliest happy memory at school?
- Did you want to have that education?
- Why didn't you have that education?
- What games did you play?
- Were you very good at games?
- Which teacher do you remember most fondly?
- Did you work while you were still at school?
- If so, what did you do?
- Did you keep all the money or give some or all to your parents?
- How old were you when you left school?

Holidays

- What were the important holidays?
- What were some of the family's traditions?
- Did you go away for holidays
- Where did you go?
- What are some of your happiest memories?

The Wars

- Did you go to war?
- What rank were you?

78

- Did you have close buddies?
- Do you ever see them or think about them?
- Were you scared/
- What do you feel about wars?

Friends

- Who is, was, or still your best friend?
- Why was or is he your best friend?
- Whom have you known the longest?
- What is your most treasured memory?

Hobbies

- What is your favorite hobby?
- When did you first take it up?
- What was your favorite sport?
- Did you get the chance to play often?
- Did you ever have time to read a lot?
- Who are your favorite authors?
- What are your favorite spectator sports?
- Who is your favorite sports figure?
- What is your favorite movie?

Politics

- What is your political affiliation?
- Has it always been the same?
- Who was the "best" president?

- Who was the "worst" president?

Greatest Challenge

- What was your greatest challenge?
- How did you meet it?

First Job

- What was your first job?
- How did you get to and from work?
- Did you like the job?
- How old were you when you got your first suit of clothes?

How Many Jobs Did You Have?

- What were the jobs?
- Why did you change?
- In which jo were you the happiest?
- Did you make any life-long friends in any of your jobs?
- Did any special boss help you?

Travel

- Where have you visited?
- Which place did you like the most?

Your Life with Mother

- When did you meet your spouse>
- Do you still remember what she looked like then?
- How old were you when you got married?

- How much money did you have then?
- Did you have to save hard?
- When did you buy your first house?
- Were you proud of it?
- What was your first car like?
- How many children did you want?
- Were you happy?

Places You have Lived

- How many have there been?
- Which did you like the most?

Disappointments in Life

- What is your greatest disappointment?
- How did you deal with it?

Achievements

- What do you feel is your greatest achievement?
- In what have you had the most pride?

Priorities

- How important was your job to you?
- How important was the family?
- Did that order change over time?

Changes

What are the major changes you have seen taking place in your lifetime?

- Technically

- Socially

- Medically

- Internationally

Most Admired Person

- Whom have you admired most?

- Why?

If You Had Your Life to Live Over Again

- What would you make any changes?

- What would they be?

Once you have the answers to the above questions (and any others you want to add), write up a brief outline of your loved one's life. Share it with him — so many memories will be shared. And share it with others in his life.

This simple collected outline will help to keep his life happy.

Personal Outline

Power of Music

by Lois J. McCloskey

The power of music has been known — yet not fully understood — to humans in all times and in all cultures. Music is a means of expressions, music connects emotions—hope, regret, love — and our stories. As a form of communication, music connects us with other human beings, our inner spirits, and our history in a way that words alone cannot. Music is the human language that bridges cultures, genders, and generations.

The power of music grows as we age. To the elderly, music can be a vehicle of reminiscence, such as when an old song brings back the vivid memory of an experience in the distant past—a memory resplendent with not only the story, but the senses and the mood. Our memories are imprinted with music. Music helps us all to define our lives: songs symbolize an era of our life, bring us together in community, and for some become a form of prayer. As one elder said, "Music is emotion from another time. It shapes our personal landscape."

When words alone make little sense, music becomes an effective means of communication. Aging and disease can leave the body with physical and cognitive disabilities which make expression difficult. Elders with memory loss brought on by conditions such as Alzheimer's disease often lose the ability to verbalize their thoughts and feelings and to understand the messages spoken to them. Awareness for these elders moves to a different, more intuitive plane where tone of the voice and body language speak more loudly. Music speaks to them and for them, and helps them bring clarity to their thoughts and experience. For them, the emotions and spirit that music conveys transcend the spoken word. In some cases, these individuals no longer speak, but they sing!

During a hearing of the U.S. Senate Special Committee on Aging, the well-known neurologist and author Oliver Sacks, M.D. testified that "many elderly patients with strokes are aphasic, they have lost some of their ability to articulate or use words; but the words that are lost may come back with singing… "Musician/singer/actor Theodore Bikel stated, "Human beings are in need of music—not as frill and luxury but as a basic necessity."

Music and memory are long-time companions who are well suited to one another. Using music as a catalyst, reminiscing can promote well-being and self-esteem, paving the way toward good spiritual and mental health.

Music may be a helpful a tool and beneficial for a person with memory loss, but there are definite things to keep in mind:

- Music must be relevant to the person you are working with, i.e. they may have sung in a church choir, so hymns may be music they relate to. Musical tastes are individual and vary. Find out what a person likes or has listened to in the past.

- Not all people are group participants. People with memory lass may begin to become more isolated and do not wish to socialize or to be a part of a group.

- Music programs need to be individual as well as group functions.

- Avoid overstimulation. Sometimes people can become agitated by music that is too fast or too loud. Generally, slower tempos and more melodic music works better. (i.e. Strauss waltzes).

- Don't have music on continuously. Have periods of quiet.

- Music may be incorporated into the daily routine.

- For bathing: Choosing music that's relaxing and something the individual enjoys may make bathing a more enjoyable experience.

- Before meals: Turn music down or off during meals, because it may direct the person's attention away from eating.

- Massage: Putting quiet music on and giving hand massage is noninvasive and nonthreatening, and is also relaxing.

- Exercise to music.

- Reminiscing with music may tap into long-term memory.

- Have a portable tape or CD player in the person's room, so when they lie down for rest in the day, or sleep at night, they have access to some relaxing music.

- Use of various instruments such as a portable electronic keyboard, autoharp, or guitar may be used to engage people by making them strum, touch, or make sounds on various instruments.

- Using the human voice and singing to people informally while they are dressing or performing other such activities of daily living may be helpful to motivate or to distract.

- Music is the most social of the arts, and a person doesn't have to be particularly musical to participate. A person in the late stages of Alzheimer's disease may still respond to music. It is a valuable tool to use when people are dying, and may be beneficial in assisting with pain management by helping to foster relaxation.

It has been said that **"music is the universal language."** In order to learn the "language," one must use imagination and creativity. The aforementioned are suggestions and ideas which may be tailored to fit individual situations.

"There is no better time than now.
The time to live is now.
The time to dream is now.
The to imagine and
forget the past is now.
The time to shine is now.
The time to bleed, sweat, and
determine yourself for the
things you want most is now."

Anonymous

Caregiving for the Elderly

One of the most dramatic successes of modern life has been the increase in life expectancy. With profound decreases in child and adult morality, most people can expect to grow old. For the majority, the "golden years" are just that—a time during which they can enjoy the fruits of their lifetime labors. However, a substantial minority of older people develop chronic illnesses and disabilities, for which they require regular assistance.

What is Caregiving

Caregiving, simply, is the regular provision of care to someone. The nature of care depends on the specific needs of the recipient. A frail older person, for example, may need help with household tasks such as cleaning, preparing meals, and arranging medical services or transportation. Those who are more disabled may need assistance with daily living activities such as dressing, bathing, or toileting. Older people with memory deficits due to Alzheimer's disease or similar disorders require help with though t— related tasks: making decisions, managing money, and getting from place to place. Older people receiving care also have emotional needs as a natural consequence of chronic disability; they may become fearful, depressed or angry. At times, they may take these feelings out on the people closest to them — their caregivers.

Who are Caregivers?

It has been estimated that between 5.8 – 7 million people in the country provide regular assistance to a frail older person. Family caregivers are a varied group. Many are husbands or wives of the older person and are, themselves, often limited in the activities they can perform. Another large group of caregivers are the children of older people, particularly daughters and daughters-in-law, and, on occasion, sons. Caregivers also include other relatives — sister and brothers, nieces, nephews, cousins and grandchildren — as well as friends and acquaintances. As a whole, family members traditionally have provided about 80% of homecare for the impaired elderly. Involvement in assisting the frail elderly can range from a few minutes a day to around-the-clock care.

In most families, one person becomes the primary caregiver, usually the individual who has the most responsibility for organizing and providing assistance to the care recipient. Primary caregivers usually bear more of the burden of providing care, but they also have the greatest say over how things are done.

Secondary caregivers are other relatives or friends who lend, or who could potentially lend, additional assistance.

Stresses and Rewards of Caregiving

While families have always helped their elders, both the number of people needing assistance and the amount of help they require is unprecedented. As a consequence, the demands and stresses of caregiving can become difficult to manage and, on occasion, may become overwhelming.

Caregiving is a job, with tasks, responsibilities and the potential for stresses and rewards. Caregivers can function best at their jobs if they can prepare by learning about their relative's condition and about the strategies for care and care alternatives available to them. Professionals working with family caregiving offers, fulfilling a sense of obligation and returning the affection and caring offers, fulfilling a sense of obligation and returning the affection and caring they may have received over the years.

Like any other stressful situation, caregiving can have adverse consequences for the caregiver's own physical or emotional health. The physical demands on caregivers can exacerbate health problems or make them vulnerable to new illnesses and problems. The emotional demands of caregiving can be considerable, resulting in feelings of sadness, depression, anxiety or anger. Research has found that as many as 40% of caregivers experience significant symptoms of depression. Anger is another common emotion, whether resulting from the care recipient's behavior, the absence of a relative's help, or the feeling of entrapment in the situation. Decreased social activity and impaired functional status are frequently reported.

Is it useful to distinguish between direct effects and ripple effects when considering caregiver stresses/ Direct effects are the stresses resulting from providing assistance directly to the older person. Care tasks such as bathing or dressing may be physically difficult for the caretaker to perform, and the amount of care needed may be exhausting or time consuming. Furthermore, care can be emotionally draining, particularly when the recipient is emotionally draining, particularly when the recipient is emotionally upset or difficult to manage due to memory loss. Ripple effects, on the other hand, are the consequences of caregiving on other parts of the caregiver's life. Caregivers may feel torn between responsibilities to the care recipient and to other family members; they may have to relinquish retirement plans, work, friendships, or other personal interests or activities. For many people, these ripple effects are more difficult and stressful than their actual care activities.

While any caregiving situation can be stressful, particular groups of caregivers have special concerns.

Only children, for example, often must assume alone all the responsibilities for their parents. Another group includes caregivers who must balance employment with caregiving, coping with competing demands from work, caregiving and their other family and social obligations, often without the time and energy to meet all of these responsibilities. Husbands or wives in a second marriage must confront the potential for misunderstandings between step-parents and step-children about financial arrangements and care provision. Finally, another special group of caregivers are those individuals who, in addition to aiding an older relative, are also caring for another disabled family member.

However, not everything associated with caregiving is stressful. Many caregivers gain a sense of satisfaction from a job well done, or because they are fulfilling their duty or obligation to the care recipient. Support and encouragement from other people can also buffer the caregiver from stress. Research has shown repeatedly that receiving emotional support from family and friends provides an important buffer the caregiver from stress. Research has shown repeatedly that receiving emotional support from family and friends provides an important buffer against the stress and burden of caregiving. It is the social contact, more than any tangible care they may provide that is important. Sharing information about the patient's condition and the disease can help to bring family more into play. Use of professionals (physicians, nurses, clergy) to draw the family into more supportive positions can be effective.

Finally, an important part of being a good caregiver is taking care of one's self. Although many caregivers have described themselves as feeling both physically and emotionally better as the result of successfully managing caregiving challenges, many also feel overwhelmed. Feelings of emotional distress or physical symptoms should be viewed as signals that caregivers need to take better care of themselves. This will benefit caregiver and care recipient alike.

Getting help

Various sources of information exist to help families learn more about their relative's condition and about different ways of providing care.

With this information, families can be better prepared for the everyday issues they control, as well as for the stresses that lie ahead. At least several kinds of help are useful for families taking care of their chronically ill relatives: information, support groups, counseling, legal and financial planning, and services programs.

Information

Many books about caregiving or care of people with specific disabilities such as Alzheimer's disease and other dementing illness have been written in recent years, and can be found in bookstores and public libraries. National associations for particular disease or their local chapters are also good sources of information. The blue pages of the telephone directory can help families get in contact with these organizations. Primary care physicians and nurses are also an important information resource.

Support Groups

Support groups are another good resource for caregivers. Th these groups, families share with one another the information they have found useful in caring for their loved one and provide comfort by sharing experiences and solutions to specific disease, or on the general issue of caregiving; they may be run by professionals.

Counseling

For some caregivers, counseling from a trained mental health professional knowledgeable about issues of aging can be very useful. Counseling is particularly helpful for caregivers who find themselves under a lot of stress, or who feel they need some time to sort out the directions they want to go. The counselor may want to invite other family members to counseling sessions or to hold a family meeting as a way of increasing mutual understanding of the situation, leading to a plan in which everyone pitches in to provide some help.

Legal and Financial Planning

Another important step for caregivers is to learn about the legal and financial aspects of their situation. Families need to consider how they can meet the costs of long-term care without becoming impoverished. If the care recipient has a dementing illness and is likely to become incompetent, legal steps will need to be taken to authorize someone else to make that person's financial and health care decisions. Information about legal and financial issues of care may be available through support groups, or through legal services, attorneys and financial planners.

Service Programs

A very important part of getting help is to identify programs which provide assistance in caring for the older person. **Day centers**, an important resource, are now available in many communities, and help both the caregiver and care recipient. Day centers help the caregiver by taking care of the older person during the day and help the participant by providing stimulating activity and an opportunity to interact with others. A good day center can play an important role in maintaining the functioning and well-being of older, disabled individuals.

In respite care a nurse's aide or other trained person provides help in the older person's home, relieving the caregiver for a period of time to give the primary caregiver a break. Home health care is available to meet specific needs, including skilled care, personal care and homemaker chore care.

While families may be reluctant to consider institutional care, it may become necessary if the care needs of the older person become too great for the family to manage. For caregiver's assisting a seriously disabled person, especially when the person's condition is deteriorating, its is important to give consideration to long-term care, including residential and nursing home care. The decision to place a person in a 24-houir care facility is one of the most difficult faced by caregivers, but when the demands being placed upon them become more that they can handle, it may be time to consider placement. As with most difficult decisions, it is better to investigate options and make plans before a crisis point is searched, for in some areas, care facilities will have long waiting lists.

For more information about the types of services available in a particular community, contact local support groups, area agencies on aging or the blue pages of the telephone directory.

Developed by Mental Disorders of the Aging Research Branch, National Institute of Mental Health, 5600 Fishers Lane, Room 7-103, Rockville, MD 20857.

"Patience and perseverance have a magical affect before which difficulties disappear and obstacles vanish."

John Quincy Adams

Depression in the Elderly

Throughout our lifetimes, emotions play a vital role. The richness and complexity of our emotions are part of what make us distinctly human. They effect how we see and interact with our world and, at the same time, they are responsive to the events around us. Since ancient times, scientists and philosophers have tried to understand the causes of our emotions. Why, for example, should two people have distinctly differing emotional reactions to the same situation? Ancients would have said that differing emotional reactions to the same situation were the result of "humours" or bodily fluids. Today, we know that some feelings and reactions are normal and healthy parts of living; other feeling, however, may signal a problem that requires evaluation and treatment by a competent mental health professional. Depression is one of those common emotions that affects people of all ages, and sometimes requires the benefits from professional help.

What is depression?

The concept of depression has at least two very different meanings. It refers both to an often-felt normal emotion of sadness to a diagnosable and treatable mental health problem. We know that almost everyone of every age occasionally suffers from brief experiences of "the blues" or sadness. These feelings are normal. Feelings of grief or bereavement, too, may be quite normal when a loss has occurred. However, when these feelings occur again and again, last for several weeks or months without a let-up, and interfere in an important way with everyday activities, the feelings could indicate the presence of what mental health professionals call "depressive illness," or "clinical depression."

Depressive illness can occur at any age. Studies have found that among the elderly in institution s— long-term care and acute care facilities alike — the prevalence of medically significant clinical depression is as high as 10-20 percent. In the community, however, clinical depression in those over 65 years of age is a present in perhaps one to two percent of the population, a lower rate than found in younger populations. Yet, research also has found that over 10 percent of the elderly living in the community, while not suffering from depressive illness per se, may be affected by important and treatable symptoms of depression associated with physical illness, life changes, or stress.

In the elderly, depressive illness can take several forms and is sometimes difficult to recognize. Depressive illness may be masked by physical complaints, be hidden by the sufferer from family and friends, or be misperceived as a normal part of aging. Yet, it is important to remember that depressive illness generally is treatable. Neither depressive illness that itself nor the act of seeking treatment for the illness is indicative of a character weakness or personality flaw. Depressive illness is just that, an illness able to be treated or cured, if the prudent decision to seek treatment is made. No one need suffer needlessly from untreated severe depression

What causes depressive illness?

While the precise mechanism through which depression occurs has not yet been discovered, usually, a number of factors — based within the person's biology and environment — combine to bring about depression. Each person's reactions depends on how those factors affect him or her personally. Some people have an inborn tendency toward depression. However, that doesn't mean that they are more automatically going to have a depressive illness; it means only that they are more likely to have one. Depending on their personality development and life experiences, they may escape severe depression altogether. A prior history of depression, too, may make depression a more likely, but not necessarily inevitable, occurrence in older persons.

It is also not surprising that a person subjected to a continuing series of severe personal losses may develop depressive illness. Events, such as the deaths or other loss of loved ones and companions, chronic physical illnesses, unexpected or continuing financial problems, or severe changes in life-style can combine to create terrible suffering and loss of self-esteem, leading to depressive illness.

Physical illness, too, has been shown to play a role in depression of later life. Depression may accompany chronic health problems in particular. Increased physical disability may predispose a person to depression, heighten the risk of suicide, and increase the likelihood of recurrent depressive episodes.

Depressive symptoms may appear as a side-effect of the use of certain prescription and over-the-counter medications used to treat physical disorders. In particular, many elderly people being treated for age-related illnesses are given medicines that, while effective in combating the physical problem, can affect the emotions. Certain blood pressure medication, for example, may cause depression as an immediate or long-term side0effect. When several medications are being used at the same time, the combination of the medicines can cause mood changes. Thus, it is important for physicians to know of all medications being prescribed and over- the-counter medicines being used to help either diagnose or prevent a depression that is a side-effect of medication.

Yet, despite our ability to identify factors that may increase the likelihood of depression, spontaneous depression in later life may occur for the first time with no apparent causes. Indeed, the most severe melancholic depressions (in which patients lose interest in virtually all activities of living) are prone to sudden onset.

Recognizing depressive illness

Depression affects a person's physical well-being, feelings, thoughts, behavior with others, and general ability to function. Depressed people demonstrate an overall loss of interest or pleasure in their usual activities and often appear sad, apathetic, and withdrawn from others. They may act tearful, agitated, angry, or irritable. They often talk of feelings of guilt, worthlessness, or hopelessness. Frequently they exhibit loss of appetite and subsequent weight loss, have trouble sleeping, and appear tired. When symptoms such as these are not brief, or if brief, tend to recur, professional advice should be sought.

Sometimes, depressed older persons will complain of aches and pains throughout the body or of fears of symptoms they believe are signs of serve physical illness. At times, it is difficult to figure out which symptoms are based on a physical problem and which are based on emotions. Vague complaints that have no true physical basis may be indicative of an underlying depression, a determination that can be made only by a competent treating professional.

In other cases, older persons are considered "senile" or thought to be suffering from Alzheimer's disease, when they actually are suffering from severe depression. In such cases of what physicians call "pseudodementia," memory seems to fade; complicated thinking seems difficult. They seem to have trouble with concentration. In such cases, it is important for a qualified mental health practitioner who specializes in treatment of the elderly to ensure that so-called "senility" is not a treatable, reversible depression in disguise.

On occasion, true memory loss (or dementia) may coexist with depression. In this case, treating the depression will not improve the memory deficits experienced, but such treatment will improve the patients' quality of life, enabling them to cope more successfully with their memory impairment.

The safest way to manage any of these apparent symptoms of depression is to seek professional care. Self-diagnosis, particularly in the elderly in the elderly for whom depression may be a symptom of an age-specific physical disorder, is dangerous.

Seeking treatment

While depression is usually a self-limiting condition, with most patients experiencing spontaneous recovery or marked improvement, it is dangerous to take a "wait and see" approach when dealing with elderly. Depression itself can cause physical problems in the older adult. For example, a depressed older person may lose interest in food, become malnourished, and, thus, weaken the body's resistance to disease. Because depressive illness frequently distorts judgement, a depressed person may ignore rashes, changes in stool or urine, or other signs of a physical illness in need of treatment. Moreover, the risk of suicide among the depressed elderly is significant, especially among those living alone and already physically ill. Thus, when an older person complains of being depressed or not caring, when that person evidences persistent changes in behavior, evaluation by a mental health professional is important.

Outpatient mental health evaluations can be obtained at mental health clinics or from independent mental health professionals with offices in the community. Community mental health centers—publicity-funded mental health clinics — exist in most areas and usually maintain graduated fee schedules. Whether evaluation and treatment is sought at a clinic or from a private practitioner, it is advantageous to see an individual who is familiar with problems of the elderly.

Frequently, local Area Agencies on Aging, local or county offices of mental health professional societies can provide guidance in locating high-quality professional help. Older persons seeking mental health evaluation may wish to seek a referral from their own doctor.

An evaluation for depression typically includes a determination of whether a biological condition of medications in use are implicated in the depressive symptoms in question. The older person and any accompanying concerned other will be asked about both the kind, severity, frequency, duration, and past history of depressive symptoms, and about any past or current life circumstances that may have precipitated or contributed to the current symptoms of an apparent depression.

If a finding is made that the older individual is suffering from a depressive illness, a number of specific treatments are available. The type of treatment recommended by the treating professional is made on the basis of detailed information about the nature of the depression itself, the course of the illness, the family history, and the response to previous treatment.

Research has shown that, as in other age groups, the elderly often respond quickly to therapy. Some therapy methods include family members; others involve small groups; and still others involve only the depressed person and a mental health professional. Antidepressant medications frequently are prescribed by a psychiatrist or other treating physician for people with more serious depression, unless medical reasons preclude their use. Such medications in treating many cases of severe depressive illness over time when used in the hands of careful and especially physicians.

Treatment outcome

Scientific studies have shown that 60-80% of depressed elderly outpatients can be treated effectivity with psychotherapy and/or with antidepressant medication. The remaining patients frequently benefit from more specialized forms of psychiatric care, sometimes provided in the hospital. Some patients may need to remain on medication to prevent recurrence, a situation similar to taking medication on an ongoing basis for high blood pressure or diabetes.

Can depression occur again? Unless steps are taken to prevent recurrence, the answer is probably yes. Depression is a recurrent illness; most individuals, if followed long enough, suffer new episodes. Early relapse is associated with patients who either have had a substantial number of prior episodes or who suffer a first episode late in life. The elderly generally are at greatest risk for recurrence. That is why understanding what caused the initial depression and taking appropriate early action is so important. Depression treated early have a better chance of a successful outcome.

Moreover, a stable personal environment will decrease the risk of further depressive episodes. Close personal ties and an intact social network provide the patient with personal support and help the clinician monitor patient progress. This support may come from family and friends and may be strengthened further by social services service agencies and mental health centers. The presence of sufficient service agencies and mental health centers. The presence of sufficient service may make the difference between a life at home or in a hospital.

In sum

Depressive illness — a medically significant disorder — does not respect age. Equally, effective treatment of this illness transcends the age of the patient. When depression occurs in the elderly, it should not be confused with either natural aging or with other age-specific illnesses. Depression, whether an underlying cause of a physical complaint, as a consequence of a physical disorder, or as a spontaneously occurring primary illness, can be readily diagnosed and treated by a component mental health professional who is especially attuned to the mental health needs of the elderly. Local health and social service agencies, health professional societies, and other health care organizations can help locate appropriate professional help. With that treatment, depressive illness, in fact, can be cured.

Developed by Mental Disorders of the Aging Research Branch, National Institute of Mental Health, 5600 Fishers Lane, Room 7-103, Rockville, MD 20857.

"To love and be loved
is to feel the sun
from both sides."

David Viscott

Bereavement in the Elderly

Bereavement, the human response to the loss of another to whom one is deeply attached, is a normal and inevitable experience that we all face at some time in our lives. The likelihood of experiencing this strong emotional event increases as we age and lose our family and friends. For most people, the grief associated with bereavement diminishes over time, particularly with active work on our part and on the part of others close to us. However, for perhaps 15-20% of us, the process does not subside on its own; rather, it remains unresolved as a source of counting distress and maladjustment. When this occurs, recovery may be facilitated by intervention from mental health professionals and other counselors.

This fact sheet describes the normal course of bereavement, as well as the potential complications of the process. It identifies factors that may encourage resolution of the grief and mourning that company bereavement.

What is bereavement?

Bereavement is the process through which a person expresses the grief and other strong emotions associated with the death of a loved one. For the older person, this process most frequently is triggered by the death of a spouse, sibling or adult child. Scientists and mental health professionals today understand bereavement as an emotional outpouring resulting from why is called separation distress, a constellation of feelings associated with profound loss.

The experience of separation distress acutely disrupts a person's normal biological and emotional balance; yet, separation distress is both normal and appropriate when a loved one has died. It allows both positive and negative emotions to be vented. For example, grieving — one of the strongest feelings associated with separation distress — may have a profound effect on the conduct of daily life. Grief may be expressed by pangs of yearning for the person who has died, crying, sorrowful mood, disruption of sleep, loss of appetite, apathy, fears, anxiety, preoccupation with objects and locations associated with the deceased, illusory experiences, vivid dreams of the person who has died, tactile or visual hallucinations, and multiple physiological symptoms and ailments.

Scientists believe that some of these manifestations of separation distress are thought to reflect the tendency of the bereaved person to search for what has been lost. Why would a bereaved survivor search for the lost person? Equally, and perhaps more fundamentally, why is the pain and suffering of bereavement necessary to a person's ultimate health and well-being? The answer lies in the fact that a social animals, we experience such losses profoundly. This separation response — bereavement — foster the reestablishment of protective bonds in the circumstances of separation, and occurs even if irrevocable loss through death is the cause of the separation.

Is bereavement the same for everyone?

The course of grief varies from person to person. Forty percent of us will experience the most intense distress within a few months after a loss; by the fifth or sixth month, our grief will begin to abate. Perhaps another 25% of us will experience intense separation distress throughout the whole first year after our loss. About a third will never manifest severe separation distress at any time during acute bereavement. For a small group of bereaved persons, separation distress is delayed by as much as three to six months after the loss. Still, in the average person, grief remains moderately intense for at least one year after a death.

The course of bereavement refers specifically to the emotional distress caused by the death of a loved one. It does not refer to the social readjustments that accompany the loss. Yet, these interpersonal accommodations and alterations in life patterns made se the result of the death are stressful in and of themselves and should not be minimized. The need to learn new skills such as home management, meal preparation, person may occupy the survivor for up to two years or more after he loss.

It is not uncommon to hear a newly bereaved individual ask "When do you get over it?" Unfortunately, the answer is not simple. As noted earlier, each person works through the experience of bereavement individually. Certainly, no one forgets the person who has died; to do so would probably not be desirable. However, over time, the ability to remember that person without profound grief generally improves substantially over the first year. The social readjustment to a new life-style likely will be well under way through the second year. Some will take longer, and some will take less time than the rough guideposts described here.

Complicated bereavement

The most common medically relevant complication of bereavement occurs in cases of unresolved or chronic grief. In such cases, separation distress does not subside over a reasonable period of time. The grief continues at a high level of intensity, disrupting both the ability to function as parents, workers and friend sand the capacity to enjoy life itself. Chronic grief may occur either when separation distress is delayed, or when manifestations of early separation distress do not subside. It is also associated with symptoms of major depressive illness, panic attacks and generalized anxiety disorders, described in other fact sheets in this series. When this unremitting pattern of grief becomes conspicuous, it is wise to seek expert help. Both evaluation and support are available from certified skilled counselors, including members of bereavement self-help organizations, clergy and mental health professionals.

The resolution of grief

No one single prescription can simply resolve grief. Because bereavement is a process that must be completed, the resolution of grief takes time. However, a number of positive factors affect the duration of grieving. First, when the death has occurred, we should trust our individual judgements about what is right for us. Decisions need not be rushed; friends often are willing to provide a nonjudgemental sounding board. Very few decisions irrevocable, and major decisions, such as the sale of a home or a move, should be postponed for a time. A planned, problem-solving approach often helps resolve both emotional and practical problems encountered at this time.

Working through grief takes time; pacing helps provide both a respite form and ability to balance emotional demands. Grief should neither be rushed nor avoided. Sources of family and social support may be able to provide specific devise about what to expect and how to manage feelings such as loneliness. Typically, we turn to family members early on; later, we may become involved in new social groups that share interests or provide support.

Professional evaluation and help are available for those of us who may not think we are managing well on our own. Such counseling may serve to reassure us that we, indeed, are coping well. If other treatment is needed, psychotherapy ("talking" therapy) or medications may be recommended. Neither should be feared. Treatment of what may have become a crippling depression may well alleviate further unnecessary suffering.

While the availability and type of supportive resources vary from community to community, many areas have special groups for the recently bereaved. Our need for services are as varied as are our methods of managing the grieving process itself. No one method may be best for each of us. Information about such groups can be found by contacting the local Department of Health, family services agency or church.

Developed by Mental Disorders of the Aging Research Branch, National Institute of Mental Health, 5600 Fishers Lane, Room 7-103, Rockville, MD 20857.

10 WARNING SIGNS OF CAREGIVER STRESS

j. DENIAL – about the disease and its effect on the person who's been diagnosed. I know mom's going to get better.

k. ANGER – at the person with Alzheimer's or others: that no effective treatments or cures currently exist, and that people don't understand what's going on. If he asks me that question one more time I'll scream!

l. SOCIAL WITHDRAWAL – from friends and activities that once brought pleasure. I don't care about getting together with the neighbors anymore.

m. ANXIETY – about facing another day and what the future holds. What happens when he needs more care than I can provide?

n. DEPRESSION – begins to break your spirit and affects your ability to cope. I don't care anymore.

o. EXHAUSTION – makes it nearly impossible to complete necessary daily tasks. I'm too tired for this.

p. SLEEPLESNESS – caused by a never-ending list of concerns. What if she wanders out of the house or falls and hurts herself?

q. IRRITABILITY – leads to moodiness and triggers negative responses and reactions. Leave me alone!

r. LACK OF CONCENTRATION – makes it difficult to perform familiar tasks. I was so busy, I forgot we had an appointment.

s.   HEALTH PROBLEMS – begin to take their toll, both mentally and physically. I can't remember the last time I felt good.

Pass this on to a Caregiver you know!

Reprinted from: Alzheimer's Disease and Related Disorders Association, Inc.
919 N. Michigan Avenue, Suite 1100, Chicago, IL 60611. – 1676
(800) 272-3900 • www.Alz.org.

Help for the Caregiver

It's a typical scenario: You start by caring for your parent, spouse, or sibling an hour here, an hour there. But once your loved one's Alzheimer's disease has progressed beyond the initial stages, that's no longer possible. Pretty soon, you are devoting full-time to watching over your patient. Presto — you've become an around-the-clock caregiver!

Most often, the progress of Alzheimer's disease requires significant changes to the family's schedule and commitments. A caregiver trying to do most of the work alone will soon find it an impossible task. Even with several caregivers taking turns, it's not uncommon for everyone to feel frustrated, depressed, and despairing. Generally, when these feelings get out of hand, it means that something ought to be done to make care a more manageable process for all concerned.

The emotional stress of watching your loved one go downhill cannot be overestimated. Do not be ashamed or embarrassed to seek relief. Even the physical demands can be exhausting. Lifting, bathing, dressing, toileting, and feeding your loved one must be performed carefully in order to prevent injuries to both your loved one and yourself. However, when you get pressed for time, trying to care for your loved one and your household, being careful could easily become the last thing on your mind.

Sooner or later, caregivers realize they need help. But where do you look?

To get started, it is suggested that you make contact with a social worker connected to your local hospital, country or state agency on aging, or local religious or charitable organizations. You can find these in your yellow pages

113

under "social services" or "human services." Another route to pursue is your local department of health. These agencies can help you with financial advice, assistance with tax or Medicare forms, locating special-needs housing, and services that provide transportation and meals.

What are the sources of information about available services?

The Eldercare Locator is a nation-wide service to help families and friends find information about community services for older people. The Eldercare Locator gives you access to an extensive network of organizations serving older people at state and local community levels. The Eldercare Locator can connect you to information sources for a variety of services including:

- home delivered meals

- transportation

- legal assistance

- housing options

- recreation and social activities

- adult day care

- senior center programs

- elder abuse prevention

- nursing home ombudsman

Occasional Needs

If you already spend most of your time at home, you may wish to have someone step-in so you can rub errands — or simply take a much-needed rest. In many areas, volunteers organized by religious, local government, or community groups will step-in for a few hours. Adult day-care programs offering personal care, meals, recreational activities, and some therapies should be available for short and long periods. Not all of these are expensive — often churches, synagogues, YMCAs, and hospitals run such programs on a sliding scale, based on your ability to pay. You may even find one that's free!

Part-and Full-Time Help

If you need more than occasional help, you may want to look into hiring a health care aide to come to your home on a regular basis. These aides can bathe, dress, and feed the patient, administer medications, and even shop, cook, and do light housework.

Aides can be hired directly or through an agency. The advantages of hiring one yourself are that you have greater control over who you choose — you do the interviewing, screening, and you pay them directly (no add-on fee from agency). The biggest disadvantage is that, if the person doesn't work out or fails to show up one day, you're stuck with no help. Home health agencies spare you the search and much of the hassle. They're also equipped to send you replacement aide immediately.

In the later stages of the patient's Alzheimer's, you might consider a hospice program, which can take place in your home or in a nursing facility. Hospice programs are designed primarily to manage (ease) the patient's pain to help patient and caregiver cope with impending death. Home hospice care can Home hospice care can be given by a visiting nurse, social worker, home health aide, clergy, and volunteers. Durable medical equipment like hospital beds, medical supplies such as incontinent pads, and medications are also covered in such a plan. The National Hospice Helpline at 1-800-658-8898 can give you information on hospice locations in your area.

Institutional care ranges from residence centers for ambulatory patients who need only limited assistance to nursing homes for bed-bound patients who need only limited assistance to nursing homes for bed-bound patients with continual needs. Your agency on aging should have a list of licensed facilities. It is recommended that you visit several facilities to see how staff interacts with patients. You may want to make a point of coming during visiting hours so you can talk to residents and their family members and see how they like the facility. (Another suggestion: If you like what you see during the day, come back one night to see if the night staffing is adequate to meet the needs of all patients.)

Help for you

The person most often overlooked in the caring process is the caregiver. It is critical not to neglect your own needs. You'll be a less effective caregiver in the long run if you cannot admit your own limitations and play to your strengths.

Here are few tips:

- Learn as much as you can about your loved one's medical condition up front, so you know what to expect and can anticipate problems. You'll be better equipped to organize the home environment and set up a routine to minimize disruption and maximize the quality of family life for all members.

- **Don't try to play the martyr and take everything on yourself.** Let other family and friends know that you can't do it without their help. You're not doing the Alzheimer's patient or your family any favors by trying to isolate them from one another. Get a commitment from all family members to contribute to the care in whatever ways they can. This begins with a firm, spoken consensus that you are all in this together, and that you all agree on the best course of action. Decisions that are unanimous — or as nearly unanimous as is humanly possible — spread the responsibility among family members more equally.

- **Get appropriate legal and financial advice from the start.** Make sure every detail is nailed down, so you can concentrate on the important business of caregiving.

- **Seek out other caregivers for information, comfort, and a "reality check."** Look for a caregiver support group, which can provide you with much needed emotional support, as well as help in finding the right resources.

- **Make sure you get regular breaks to restore your energy and sense of self, so you can better carry out your duties as caregiver.** Allow yourself the time to do whatever it is you like to do. You should also consider taking a vacation, even if it's only for a few days. Hire a home health aide to cover for the times you're gone.

- **Accept changes in the patient's behavior.** Your control of the caregiving situation will be frequently challenged. Remember to simplify, reassure, and reinforce things for the patient.

• **Use your body wisely.** To prevent back injuries, never bend at the waist to pick up or move the patient. Instead, flex at the knees and hips and push up using the upper leg muscles. Try to work at waist level as much as you can. When transferring the patient from bed to chair, point your feet in the direction of the move; this prevents the twisting of your spine, a potentially hazardous movement.

• **If you have to put your loved one in a nursing home, try not to feel unduly guilty.** You've done everything in your power for your loved one, and it is no longer enough. Thousands of families with a loved one who has Alzheimer's have made this wrenching decision.

• **Try to keep your pleasures in your life while you are a caregiver.** Research shows that a healthy leisure life can buffer the effects of stress. Try to arrange to have some time to pursue your hobbies, spend time with a friend, go out to dinner with a loved one, or just plain read a book. You are entitled and it's good for you. Being a caregiver does not mean that you should give up things you enjoy. If you make a point of doing things you enjoy, you will be a happier and more content person.

Resource for the Caregiver

Wendy Lustbader has produced a DVD (60 minutes) on caregiving entitled: *A Prescription for Caregivers.* Filmed in front of a live audience of caregivers, the presentation is packed with humor and stories from real life. Topics include: heeding resentment as a warning sign of doing too much, the many varieties of guilt, options for self-care, and figuring out how much care is "enough." Both caregivers and professionals who assists them will find ideas on how to make life better for the giver and receiver of care. The video normally sells for $85.00, but Ms. Lustbader is giving our readers a special price of $30.00 for home use only.

She is also the author of two books: *Taking Care of Aging Family Members ($16.00)* and Counting on Kindness ($14.00). To order these resources, mail your check or money order to Wendy Lustbader, P.O. Box 13487, Burton, WA 98013, telephone: 206-985-5400.

Innovative Caregiving Resources has developed a series of 13 different videos designed to provide short periods of respite time from caregiving responsibilities while providing enjoyable interaction for the care-recipient. Each video presents a simulated visit with the care-recipient with pauses, music, props and appropriate techniques to capture and maintain the attention of an individual with moderate to advanced staged Alzheimer's disease. Titles include, Gonna Do a Little Music, Remembering When, Sharing Christmas Cheer, Sharing Favorite Things, Sentimental Sing-along, A Kibitz with David, A Visit with Maria. Additionally, Innovative Caregiving Resources has videos developed specifically for the caregiver to facilitate exercise, relaxation and ideas for cooperative activities with the care-recipient. To order or to get a catalogue, contact:

Innovative Caregiving Resources

P.O Box 17809

Salt Lake City, UT 84117-0809

801-272-9806

800-249-5600

AARP Webplace on Caregiving

http://www.aarp.org/family/caregiving

This website has information on caregiving, resources, publications and links to other caregiver website.

Making the Moment Count: Leisure Activities for Caregiving Relationships – Joanne Ardolf Decker (1997). Johns Hopkins University Press, ISBN: 080185707. This book is designed to address the burden of caregiving offering ideas for short "increments" of time that can lighten the load of caregiving. It includes sections on the importance of leisure, leisure in the caregiving process, and ideas about how to use cases in each chapter.

Failure-free Activities for the Alzheimer's Patient – Carmel Sheridan (1995). Dell Books, ISBN: 0440506050: This book offers simple activities which are enjoyable for the acre-recipient and the caregivers.

Today's Caregiver Magazine

3005 Greene Street

Hollywood, FL 33020

800-829-2734

Caregiver Connections

Maintaining a good relationship with a caregiver is vital. Here are some reminders to help keep that relationship healthy and helpful.

Stay connected. Don't allow isolation to create a forum for depression, anger and helplessness. Send e-mails, make phone calls, invite small groups of friends and family to visit. Revive the art of letter writing. Join a support group. Develop your own hobbies. Become a self-styled expert on something.

Don't depend on one person. It is easy to get in the habit of relying on just one person to provide support. This contributes to the caregiver's burnout and loss of patience. Involve family members as early as possible, and share tasks. Not everyone has the ability or the talent for around-the-clock caregiving, but they may be willing to assist with particular needs. Be specific when you ask for help.

Encourage time away. If you have a caregiver, make sure he or she takes breaks. Be willing to go to an adult daycare or be cared for by others to give the caregiver time to recharge. Take a break. For a few minutes, for a day, for a week. Recharge your physical and emotional energy by getting away from the stress of care, even if only for brief periods.

Say thank you. Caregiving can be a stressful job. Expressing consideration, emotional connection, and appreciation are ways you can help your caregiver care better for you. Recognize caregiving as a way to show love and serve. Cultivate your sense of humor. It's there, even in facing a dementing illness. Look for and create opportunities to laugh.

Take care of your physical needs. Eat well-balanced meals. Improve your fluid intake. Get the rest you need. Get periodic checkups. Stay physically active. Try to involve your loved one in swimming, walking, or biking.

Where to turn? Your local area Agency on Aging can link you with resources. Also, try the Alzheimer's Association at 1-800-272-3900, Alzheimer's Disease Education and Referral Center (ADEAR) AT 1-800-438-4380, Alzheimer's Disease Sharing Care at 1-866-736-4695.

Support Service

The majority of very frail or disabled people want to continue to live at home. Feeling part of family life and the community puts a burden on the family; usually one particular family member, called the primary caregiver. If the caregiver is to cope with increasing care demands, she must have support; that support may come from a range of sources—other family members and friends, or what is known as the "formal support system."

Before caregivers are able to deploy the formal system, they must have identified their needs, either with or without the advice of a professional, know what services are available and how to access those services.

If the care-recipient is an adult, then, where feasible, she should be included in the planning process. They know what they want, but you may have a better idea of what is possible.

Some basic guidelines are presented to enable caregivers to identify which agency or professional may help and what services they provide. To meet care needs, several services may be required.

We have set out questions you may have and attempted to answer those questions, through our Question (Q) and Answer (A) format.

Homemaker and Home Health Aide Services

For many families the first hint they have that their parent or other relative is no longer able to cope adequately, without some help, is the person's inability to do shopping, cleaning, other chores and attend to some of their own personal care needs. At this stage, the service which may enable the person to function longer in the home, is what is called, the homemaker and home health aide service.

Homemaker Services

Q. What is a homemaker service?

A. It is a service which for a fee, will provide help with shopping, cooking and household chores.

Home health Aide Services

Q. Who can help if a person can no longer bathe, dress, or take medication unaided?

A. The Home Health Aide will help with this kind of care and report to the Home Health Nurse about the person's progress.

Q. Who provides the above services?

A. Homemaker-Home Health Care Agencies. Some hospitals provide these services for their discharged patients.

Q. What about charges?

A. Charges vary. In some instances, Medicare, Medicaid, or health insurance cover such services, but only under very specific, limited circumstances. Some agencies accept only persons who can pay privately; others offer a sliding scale fee.

Q. What qualifications do homemaker/home health aides have?

A. Generally they are trained in household and personal care. They work under the direction of a health professional, a nurse or a social worker.

Q. Where can I find information about these services?

A. Through community service agencies; the local Area Agency on Aging, and listing in the Telephone Yellow Pages under Health Care Services.

Q. What are some of the questions for you to ask when trying to answer the ability of the Agency to meet the needs you require to be met?
A. Is the Agency bonded and licensed?

Is the Agency a member of the Better Business Bureau or the Chamber of Commerce?

Ask for and check out the Aide's references.

Check whether the Aide is trained to perform the duties that are needed.

Inquire whether the Aide will be supervised. By whom? Know how to reach the Supervisor?

Before the Aide starts work, settle all arrangements about such things as tasks, hours, payment, transportation costs, supervision and your expectations.

Learn who will be liable if there is an accident in your home or if something is stolen.

Maintain regular contact with the Aide's supervisor. Tell her if you are not satisfied.

Chore Services
Q. What is a Chore Service?
A. This service offers help with chores around the house — heavy housekeeping, yardwork and minor repairs.

Q. Where can these services be located?
A. Check private agencies listed in the Yellow Pages. In many areas, there are community or church sponsored programs. Ask at your local social services agency or Area Agency on Aging.

Q. *What about fees?*
A. Fees will vary according to the agency, the work done, number of hours, etc. Check with the local social services agency and Area Agency on Aging to see whether financial help is available in your community.

Emergency Response Systems

Q. *What is an Emergency Response System?*
A. These systems provide contact with local authorities such as police or rescue squads, if there is an emergency.

Q. *What is the value of such a system?*
A. Where used, they can provide a greater sense of security. But the systems should never be operated in isolation. It should only be part of a care package. Batteries should be regularly checked.

Q. *Are these systems costly?*
A. The cost depends on the complexity of the system.

Q. *Where can I find information about Emergency Response System?*
A. Contact your local social services agency or Area Agency on Aging. The service may also be listed in the Yellow Pages under Emergency Alarm Systems.

Friendly Visiting

In many cases, disablement may lead to social isolation, loneliness and then on to depression. For more older people who have always liked company, a Visiting Service may help to alleviate the loneliness.

Q. *What exactly can such a service do?*
A. Churches, synagogues, the local social service agency or the Visiting Nurses' Association should have information.

Home-Delivered Meals

Home-delivered meals can keep elderly, frail and/or disabled persons out of an institution.

Q. What is a home-delivered meals service?
A. Hot, nutritious meals are brought once a day during the week to people who cannot make their own. Other arrangements generally have to be made for weekends. Provisions may be made for special diets.

Q. What is the cost?
A. Some services are free, others have to be paid for, on an ability to pay basis. Where there is a fee, charges will vary from area to area.

Q. Who provides these meals?
A. Most services are paid for and operated by voluntary organizations, such as churches, nursing homes and senior centers. Some are provided through private agencies.

Q. Where can I get information?
A. From the local Area Agency on Aging or social service agency.

Nutrition Services

Eating a good diet is fundamental to good health and maintaining strength.

Q. Where can I get information about nutrition?
A. From a doctor, a qualified nutritionist or a dietician.

Q. Are there any places where nutritious, reasonably priced meals are available for older people?
A. Congregate dining sites are located in most areas. At these sites, the person gets a hot meal and can also take

part in the socialization and activities that go on at the dining site.

Senior Citizen Centers

These centers provide a social gathering place for older people in the community.

Q. What is a Senior Center?
A. A place which provides socialization, recreation, meals, counseling and advice on financial matters.
Q. What are these centers located?

A. In churches, synagogues, housing projects and nursing homes; or they are separate facilities.

Q. How do I locate them?
A. Contact the local social service agency or the Area Agency on Aging.

Professionals

In addition to needing help from family, friends, and using social service type services, an elderly and/ or disabled person may need help from health acre professionals. Who are some of these professionals and how can they help?

The Doctor

The doctor is generally the first professional with whom the disabled person or her caregiver comes into contact. Whenever there is any feeling of unwellness or any symptom appears, the doctor should be consulted. Some people regard conditions such as failing sight, feelings of depression, incontinence, difficulty walking, increasing forgetfulness and loss of hearing as part of the aging process. Certainly there are physical changes as one ages, but many conditions can either be arrested or treated and enable the person to have a better quality of life.

The family doctor may make a diagnosis and then refer the patient on to another professional who is equipped to design a care package, based on her recommendations, to meet the person's needs. Or she may refer the patient on to a specialist.

Q. When does the family doctor usually refer a patient to a specialist?

A. When her diagnosis indicates that the patient should be seen by some doctor who specializes in the particular condition from which the patient is suffering. There are doctors who specialize in geriatric medicine, psychogeriatric medicine, urinary tract infections, rheumatism/arthritis problems, oncology (cancer), endocrine disease (e.g. diabetes) and a range of other conditions. But the family doctor should remain the key person for complete patient care. Too often o patient has too many specialists so the primary care family doctor should coordinate all patient care.

Q. Why is it essential to follow through the doctor's treatment recommendations?

A. Many conditions can in fact be successfully treated. Others can be arrested or helped. If, for example, therapy has been recommended, and the treatment is not followed through, or medications have been prescribed and the prescription not filled the condition will become worse, leaving the person more debilitated and more dependent on the caregiver.

The Case Manager

Q. What does the Case Manager do?

A. Case managers are not available in every area. Ask the doctor; check the Yellow Pages under Human Services,

County Health Nursing Service, Area Agency on Aging and the Information and Referral Services in your area.

Q. Will a fee be required?
A. Yes, most of the time. If a fee is charged, get a written statement of the fee and what services will be provided for that fee, before you actually employ the **person.** However, some social service agencies provide this service free of charge.

Home Crae Professionals

This service may have to be invoked to take the pressure off the caregiver.

Q. What is Home Care?
A. It is a range of health and supportive services, provided at home, for people who require assistance in meeting their health care needs.

Q. Which services are included?
A. Skilled nursing, physical therapy, occupational therapy and speech therapy are included. Additionally, personal care services such as help with bathing, dressing, toileting, etc. are provided.

Q. Who delivers these services?
A. Nurses, therapists and home-health aides, through a home health agency or public health department.

The Nurse

Q. What does the Nurse do?
A. The nurse's roles are multiple. First, she will visit the very frail or disabled person at home to evaluate her condition, decide what nursing care is needed, implement the doctor's medical treatment plan and monitor the patient's progress. Where feasible, the nurse discusses the care with the patient and with the family.

Additionally, the nurse can alleviate a lot anxiety by helping the caregiver to better understand the course of the disease, counsel her on coping strategies, counsel on stress management and where indicated, how to enhance communication with the care-recipient. Another very important function is showing the caregiver basic home-caring skills. Among the skills she can demonstrate are how to lift someone who is bed-bound, how to prevent bed sores, how to give injections, ow to change dressing and how to give medications. The nurse can also provide information on home nursing equipment and where it can be rented or purchased.

The Physical Therapist

Q. *What service does a Physical Therapist provide?*
A. On the basis of the doctor's medical diagnosis and recommendations, a physical therapist prepares a treatment schedule. In some cases, basic exercise are given to restore strength and movement. Rehabilitation is very important, not only from a physical point of view, but from the psychological aspect. Sometimes the care-recipient will need a lot of encouragement and help to carry through the exercise regimen. Therapy should increase independence all alleviate some of the caregiving load.

The Occupational Therapist

Q. *What is the role of the Occupational Therapist?*
A. An occupational therapist assesses the person's ability to cope with daily activities and movement. Walking aids, eating aids, bath aids and adaptations, clothing with Velcro fasteners, ramps, rails, etc. may be recommended.

The Social Worker

Q. What is the function of the Social Worker?

A. A social worker can help the family determine what kind of help they require to meet the person's needs, directing and connecting the family to personal social services and community services that can assist them. Additionally, she is trained to counsel on stress management and on more effective communication between the caregiver and care-recipient.

Certified Therapeutic Recreation Specialist (Recreation Therapist)

Q. How would I use a Certified Therapeutic Recreation Specialist (CTRS)?

A. Research has determined that recreation is an essential component for physical and mental wellness in all people, young and old, well or disabled. A CTRS can help increase functional ability as well as the ability to access and enjoy leisure activities in both care-recipients and caregivers. A CTRS can help will access one's functional abilities and needs and develop specific recreation interventions that can help people, with and without illness and disabilities, to become stronger physically, mentally, emotionally and socially. Activities can be conducted 1:1 or for an entire family. Additionally, they can help the caregiver plan some recreation experiences that might bring relief and enjoyment to the helper as well.

General Information

Q. Where will I find information about healthcare services?
A. From doctors, hospital discharge planners, local health departments, Area Agencies on Aging, nursing homes, and in the Yellow Pages under Healthcare Agencies or Nurses.

Q. What is some basic information I should have about an agency before using it?
A. In some states, such agencies must be licensed.

The agency should consult with the care-recipient's doctor and prepare a written care-plan.

Then the supervising nurse should discuss the plan and costs with the care-recipient (where feasible) and the caregiver.

Check that the agency's staff are properly trained and qualified and licensed. Additionally, determine whether they are adequately supervised and evaluated on a regular basis.

Check out the references of the agency and its staff.

Ask for a copy of the complaints procedure.

Determine how much the service will cost. Make sure the care-plan is approved by the doctor and that the agency is certified to be reimbursed through Medicare and Medicaid or your care-recipient's insurance company.

Check that the service will be available when you need and want them.

Incontinence

Urinary Incontinence

What is Urinary Incontinence

Urinary incontinence is the loss of bladder control.
This condition often occurs among people with Alzheimer's disease and other associated disorders. Urinary incontinence may be caused by health problems such as infections of the bladder or the urinary tract. It may happen because of reactions to drugs. Many of these conditions do respond to treatment. It is important to have the cause of the incontinence investigated by your care-recipient's doctor.

Possible Caregiver Reactions

Being the caregiver, you may be the one asked to help identify the cause of the incontinence, and later with professional guidance, to help manage the problem.

Because it is such a personal issue, as bodily waste is involved, this is a very sensitive issue. You may find it difficult to actually talk about the problem with your care-recipient. He may, out of embarrassment, try to pretend that it is not happening.

Diagnosis

Among questions the doctor may have are — when did you first observe the problem; whether the loss of control has become worse over time; whether this is the first indication of such a problem; whether incontinence occurs only at night or only during the day or both night and day. How often does he urinate during any one day? Is it dribbling or leakage problem; is the urine stream a strong one; does he wake up wet? Is there pain or burning or a feeling of great urgency? What about the color and odor? Is he more upset or confused since the problem first became evident? Were any changes recently made in the amount of fluid intake, in foods, in routine consumption of alcohol, coffee or tea? Does he realize that he is having 'accidents' or wetting the bed? Do you think accidents are occurring because he cannot get to the bathroom on time?

It may help the doctor make an early diagnosis of the problem if you go along equipped with some answers, at least, to some of the foregoing questions.

Treatments

Once he has diagnosed the problem, the doctor can proceed to treat the symptoms that can be helped. Actually solving the problem may take time.

It is important not to build up false expectations, in fact the prescribed treatment may work completely, not at all, or only in part. The cause of the condition may be part and parcel of the Alzheimer's disease.

Management

Your role is to manage the person's toileting so his dignity remains intact and he is as comfortable as possible. The following coping strategies may prove useful.

- Visual cues like a stick-figure, arrows or a vividly painted door, may help him locate the bathroom more easily. Use of night lights, a bedpan or commode may help avoid accidents at night.

- Making the bathroom feel secure, e.g. handrails alongside the toilet; raising the toilet seat (devices that change the height or a raised toilet seat are available).

135

- Taking the person to the bathroom at regular intervals.

It is important not to limit the person's fluid intake, except on the device of the doctor.

Special clothing, supplies and equipment can help your care-recipient feel comfortable, eliminate many accidents and save your energy. Among equipment that may be bought are adult diapers, slipcovers for chairs, washable sheets that absorb the urine but do not become cold; bed protectors, external catheters for men or pads for women. Some products are more absorbent than others.

Your doctor, nurse or pharmacist can tell you which products should work best in your care-recipient's situations. Call ABLEDATA, telephone 800-227-0216, which has information on the range and sources of products.

Instead of buying a piece of equipment, such as a commode, it may be possible to rent it.

Bowel Incontinence

What is Bowel Incontinence

Bowel incontinence is not being able to control one's bowel movements.

The problem usually manifest itself by soiling the clothing or bedding. It is quite a separate problem from urinary incontinence which is loss of bladder control. One type of incontinence can occur without the other. Fortunately for all concerned, bowel incontinence occurs less frequently than urinary incontinence. Either the patient will be aware of what is happening and be very upset about it, or not realize that he has the problem.

Among causes bowel incontinence are the progression of Alzheimer's disease, some other medical conditions, sometimes side effects from drugs, and the result of over-use of laxatives or enemas. In other cases the pain of hemorrhoids or constipation may be the cause. Changes in the diet, eating pattern or fluid intake may also to the condition.

Any onset of bowel incontinence requires checking by the person's doctor. It is important to realize that many causes do respond to treatment.

As far as the onset of the disease is concerned, the doctor may ask you to note the course of the condition over a time, to determine whether the problem is worsening. Try therefore, to record what you observe carefully. Among questions the doctor may want you to answer are — is the problem regular or more in the form of an occasional accident; when does it happen — after eating, after exercise, seemingly at any time; is this the first manifestation of the problem; what was his bowel pattern before this stage; with what frequency does the person have a problem; what are the characteristics of the stool — is it hard, soft; at first hard then soft; does diarrhea occur; what about the size, color (for instance is pus, mucus, or blood there) and odor; what kinds of food has the person been eating; when does the incontinence occur—on the way to the bathroom; anytime; were there any other changes in the person's behavior, moods, etc. when the incontinence occurred; does he seem distressed by the problem?

The doctor will also want to know what drugs your care-recipient is taking.

Treatment may be as simple as stopping the use of certain laxatives. The doctor may prescribe new drugs or changes in the diet. He may request you to monitor the results.

Regrettably in some instances the treatment may only be partly effective. In other cases nothing may work. All you can hope to do is to keep the person clean and comfortable.

Don't try to develop your own coping techniques without input from the doctor or nurse who can make proven recommendations. If you haven't one already, ask them to develop a care-plan. Among the measures they may suggest are the following.

- You may need to make some changes in his routine; for instance, he may need regular exercise regimen and the content of a well-balanced diet to meet his needs.

- Establish a definite pattern of taking the person to the bathroom.

- It is important that he feels secure in the bathroom. Equipment, such as rails on the wall alongside the commode and a raised toilet seat can help.

- Never use an over the counter stool—softener without having consulted the doctor.

If Your Efforts Do Not Work

To save yourself work, you may consider special needs clothing, supplies and equipment. Your goal is to keep your care-recipient clean and comfortable and to save yourself undue washing. Over time, the products can be costly. Therefore, you have to weigh the cost element carefully and look for supplies that meet the need, but are not necessarily the most expensive.

Some equipment or devices, as they are commonly called, that work are: grab bars alongside the toilet; handrails and adjustable toilet seats; adult briefs (diapers); pads, liners and sheets. Some sheets may be re-used, others are thrown away after one use. Your doctor or nurse may suggest what is most useful to deal with your situation. They will know where to locate the items.

Information on equipment, devices and special clothing is available from ABLEDATA, TELEPHONE 800-227-0216

If some items such as a commode can be rented, it may be less costly to rent than to purchase.

Your Feelings

It is never easy to accept that a parent is so reliant on you for such a basic need. Many caregivers feel shock, shame, even ill, at the idea of cleaning up feces. If you feel this way, you will almost certainly feel pangs of guilt. It is important to remind yourself that the problem is part of the disease of Alzheimer's. Share your feelings with a healthcare professional.

Safety in the Home

Statistically accidents in the home account for a large percentage of the total number of all injuries and death. Some injuries lead to immobility and premature dependency. It is important therefore, for family members to examine the person's environment critically to assess how the home can be made safer and what innovations or changes are required to make it is hazard-free as possible. In your overview, consider how to prevent falls, how to avoid accidental burns or accidental poisoning or injury.

Some Steps Toward Preventing Accidents

Note: the actions will vary, depending on the type of housing and furnishings; therefore the information provided, has to be general.

Inside the House

In the Bedroom

- Have a telephone installed with the emergency numbers listed plainly.

- Place the bed against the wall so it can't move, if the persons misses a step and falls against it.

- Ensure that the lamp or a light switch is reachable from the bed.

- Check that the floor is neither slippery nor covered in tatty or slippery rugs.

- See that there are not any dangling electrical cords over which one may trip.

In the Bathroom

- Ensure that the floor is non-slip.

- Handrails against the wall can provide extra support (make sure that the bars are properly installed).

- A rubber mat in the bottom of the bath or the showerstall can make the area more secure.

In the Kitchen
- Install a fire extinguisher.

- Store china, pots/pans, foodstuff on easily accessible shelves.

- Warn against climbing on chairs to reach into upper-level cupboard or to adjust or clean windows.

- Don't have mats on the floor.

In the Living Room
- Ensure the hinged-leaf tables are safe if leaned on.

- Check that unsecured bookshelves cannot topple over and crush somebody.

- Look at the individual's whole capabilities and needs. Evaluate his whole physical setting to deal with meeting those needs. The following are steps you may decide need to be taken to make the environment more disabled-friendly:

- Check that the water temperature is not so hot it could scald somebody.

- Carefully dispose of old drugs (frequently).

- Have the person wear flame-resistant clothes; eliminate clothing with loose, floppy sleeves as they may catch fire over a stove.

- Have all electric-writing checked by a professional.

- Have a fire alarm installed and make sure it is functional at all times.

- Practice exiting procedures in case of fire.

- Check all electric cords for wear and tear.

- If a fireplace is used, have the chimney cleaned regularly.

- If possible, have electric sockets positioned where they are accessible.

- See that the person wears well-fitting shoes; without laces. Be sure he knows the movements involved in getting up from the floor, should he fall.

- If a wheelchair is used, see that it functions properly.

- If a walking cane is used, have a rubber tip put on the end to stop slippage.

Especially if He is Mentally

- Identify and remove any objects that may be dangerous; cigarettes, pipes, matches; blenders; toasters, kettles; food processors; sharp knives and long-pronged forks; can-openers.

- Space heaters, electric fans may pose a threat to a very forgetful, or disoriented person.

- Pull the circuit breaker to the electric stove each night before going to bed.

- Watch that any electrical appliances are used with great care near water make sure he can use an electric razor, heater, radio, etc. in the bathroom or kitchen without coming into contact with water.

- Guard against all electrically-related injuries.

- Hide all sharp or breakable objects.

- Keep an extra key handy in case the person locks you out.

- If he has any mobility problems at all; buy him knee-length robes to prevent tripping accidents.

- Store cleaning substances out of reach

- Store alcohol out of reach

- Ask the utility company to come and advise on how to make the stove-top safe.

- Make sure that the cold water is always run into the bath or shower first.

- If an emergency alarm system is used, make sure that it is functioning as intended.

- If the person lives alone, you, another family member or a neighbor, should call (if possibly affordable), at a certain time(s) daily to ensure he is alright (calling may also serve to make him feel more secure).

- Post **emergency phone numbers** beside every telephone.

Outside the House

- Ensure that paths and porches are even and free of obstructions.

- Repair any broken steps.

- Use adequate lighting at night.

- See that tree branches are pruned above eye level.

Especially If the Person is Mentally Impaired

- If the person is mentally impaired, don't allow him access to the car, power tools, lawnmowers or anything which may lead to injury, either to him or somebody else.

In the Summer

- Try to ensure that the person drinks enough fluids.

- Keep the environment comfortably cool.

- Discourage any exhausting activity.

- See that clothing is loose-fitting and summery (cottons are cooler than synthetics).

- Watch for hyperthermia.

Summer heat is real threat to the elderly; certain health conditions may make some even more vulnerable; as may be those with weight problems (both overweight and underweight). Heat stroke or heat exhaustion are medical emergencies.

Ways of Preventing Hyperthermia

- Drinking lots of fluids.

- Wearing light-weight, loose-fitting clothing.

- Minimizing oven use.

- Avoiding strenuous activity.

- Good ventilation; keeping the place as cool as is possible.

In the Winter

- Indoor temperatures should not fall below the comfort level the person is used to (preferably around 70 degrees).

- Be alerted to the possibility that he can no longer read the thermostats.

- Know that some drugs and alcohol may pre-dispose some people to hypothermia.

- If you suspect hypothermia, call the doctor immediately.

Actions that May Be Taken to Prevent *Hypothermia*

- Keep the temperature at a livable, constant level.

- Make sure the person is warm enough.

- If you live at a distance, ask a friend or neighbor to check periodically, preferably randomly, on the temperature in the person's residence.

- Install a large print thermometer.

"Difficult times have helped me to understand better than before how infinitely rich and beautiful life is in every way and that so many things that one goes worrying about are of no importance whatsoever."

Isak Dinesen

Providing for Basic Needs

Looking after a sick or severely disabled family member can put a lot of stress on the caregiver, who has generally had little or no training in home-care.

The person needing the care generally has a range of needs — physical, emotional, social and spiritual. Sometimes the complexity of the demands is so overwhelming that caregivers don't take time to establish any sort of system which in turn leads to an even more burdensome role. They keep on, on an ad hoc basis, becoming increasingly exhausted.

A knowledge of basic home-caring procedures can be reassuring and relieve a lot of the strain.

Organizing the Nursing Environment

- Ideally,, the furniture in the patient's room should be arranged to have easy access to the bed. The furniture should include a bedside table, a comfortable chair for when he is sitting out of bed and the floor should be non-slip; preferably covered for coziness.

- The room should always be adequately heated or cooled and fresh.

- If there is not sufficient cupboard space, build a shelf to contain nursing paraphernalia — plastic bags for refuse; personal care equipment — brush, comb, toothbrush and cup, and fresh face-cloths and towels, soap, extra glasses (that cupboard or shelf will save you many trips in and out).

- Keep all medications out of the reach of the patient who has any memory impairment of confusion.

Bathing

- It the person is afraid of getting into the bath, a bath chair may help. If he prefers showering, a shower stool may be used. Always run the cold water before the hot water and mix well. A rail beside the bath or shower may help him to get back into a standing position.

- A roller-towel fastened to a secure bar can enable him to dry himself in privacy.

- If he cannot get out of bed, then he will have to be given a bed-bath. This is better managed by someone who has had training or by two people. If you do not have the help of a bath aide, ask the nurse to demonstrate how to give a bed-bath.

- Wash his hands and face several times a day to freshen the patient and wash the genital areas after toileting.

- Attend to nails immediately after bathing as they will be more pliable.

- If you notice any changes in the patient's skin, report them immediately to the nurse or doctor.

- Hair-care for a bed-bound person can be a problem. Molded plastic vinyl shampoo basins, with attached hoses which drain into a bucket, are available at drugstores and through mail-order catalogs. The equipment provides support for the neck while the hair is being washed. After thorough rinsing, to avoid scurf build-up, see that the hair is properly brushed and dried. Dry shampoo powders may also be used; but watch for scurf build-up, if it is not completely removed.

Medication Management

Enclosed with your Caregiver's Support Kit® you'll find a complimentary pill box dispenser. Note, however, that many elderly take multiple medications at various times each day. The responsibility to administer the correct medications at the proper time is perhaps the most important part of your caregiving tasks.

To help remember the proper procedure for administering medications you can refer to the following six rights!

This procedure will ensure that:

1. the **RIGHT PERSON**

2. receives the **RIGHT MEDICATION**

3. in the **RIGHT DOSE**

4. at the **RIGHT TIME**

5. via the **RIGHT METHOD/ROUTE**

6. followed by the **RIGHT CHARTING** procedures.

You don't need to worry about the right person if you only care for one person, but many caregivers have more than one person getting medications in the household. Be sure you have the right person and the right medication for that person.

Double check, even triple check, that you have the right dose prepared. This is especially important if the patient has recently seen the doctor where changes may have been prescribed. Take time to read the pharmacy label frequently. Always check the expiration date for the medications. If the medication has expired — stop —

21. Providing for Basic Needs

do not give expired medications. Call your health care professional for instructions.

The right time for medications is the time specified or prescribed on the medication label. In general, medications can be given within one hour before or after the prescribed time. For example, a medication prescribed for 4:00 p.m. can be given any where from 3:00 p.m. to 5:00 p.m. Be sure to remember any special instructions such as "must be taken with food"

The right method/route is indicated when a health professional prescribed a medication. The method is usually orally, or by mouth, but occasionally it could be in the form of a topical skin cream, patch, eye drops etc.

Finally, keep a chart record of the medications given and note any reactions or problems encountered. Tell your health care professional if you observe any negative reactions to medications as soon as possible. You can use a calendar kept for chart purposes only. There is usually enough room to write notes and reminders and it will save you having to remember everything.

How to Avoid Medication Error

Taking the wrong medications or taking medications incorrectly can have serious consequences or even be fatal. Here are some suggestions to help you and your loved one avoid harmful drug interactions, problems with dosages and other potential adverse actions.

At Home:

- Make a list of all your loved one's medications, including dosage, frequency of use, condition it is for, name of pharmacy and prescribing physician.

- Any time your loved one's medication changes, change your list.

- Keep all medications in their original containers.

- Don't chew, crush, or break capsules or tables unless so advised. You may make the medication unsafe or ineffective.

At the Hospital:
- Take your loved one's own medication list with you.

- Ask the physician the names of any new medications to be used and the reasons they are prescribed.

- Look at all medications before your loved one takes anything, if they appear different from what he/she usually takes, question why.

- Ask hospital staff to check your loved one's hospital ID bracelet before administrating medication to prevent receiving another person's medication.

- When you loved one is ready to go home, have a knowledgeable person review each medication with you. Find out what condition it treats and whether it is to be taken in addition to what you have at home for the condition or in lieu of it. Ask about possible side effects.

- Update your medication list from home as needed.

At the Doctor's Office:
- Bring a copy of your loved one's medication list on every visit.

- If your doctor offers samples, ask if the medications will interfere with any medications your loved one is using.

- Ask the drug name, how the prescription should be filled, and how often the medication should be taken.

- Ask the doctor to write the purpose for the medication on the prescription. Drug names can be "look-a-likes" when written in longhand. Having the purpose noted will help the pharmacist to double check the prescription.

- Encourage the doctor to institute electronic prescribing as a way of enhancing patient safety.

Take it to the Doctor

Better safe than sorry. Before you leave the pharmacy, compare your doctor's prescription to the label on the bottle. You might catch a deadly mistake.

Is your NAME correct on both the prescription and the medicine bottle? If you have a name such as Bob Jones or Mary Smith, ask the pharmacist to include your middle initial.

Is your NAME on the medication correct? Look carefully. Some drug names are similar.

Is the DOSAGE the same as what your doctor told you.

Are the INSTRUCTIONS understandable? Doctors and pharmacies often communicate in LATIN. For example:

Latin	Abbreviation	Meaning
ante cibum	ac	before meals
bis in die	bid	twice a day
gutta	gt	drop
hora sommi	hs	at bedtime
oculus dexter	od	right eye
per os	po	by mouth
post cibum	pc	after meals
pro re nata	prn	as needed
quaque 3 hora	q3h	every 3 hours
quaque die	qd	every day
quarter in die	qid	4 times a day
ter in die	tid	3 times a day

When traveling KEEP your medicine with you — not checked your luggage. BRING more than enough medicine for your trip. REVIEW your dosage schedule with your doctor or pharmacist before you leave and DISCUSS whether you should make allowances for changes in time zones.

Keep a list of all your medicines and dietary supplements with you.

Prescriptions
- Do not run out
- Know the pharmacy hours; including emergency arrangements.
- Always check with the pharmacist about drug mixes.
- Be very vigilant that correct doses are taken at prescribed times.

- If any unusual symptoms show up, call the doctor immediately as they may be due to a sudden allergic reaction to some drug or due to the drug reacting negatively with some food.

Diet

- It is important to maintain a good nutritional diet.

- Present food is as attractive a manner as time and energy permit.

- Foe some patients, several small meals may be better that three larger meals (check with the doctor before making any changes).

Exercise

- There are exercises suitable for even chairbound and bedbound people. Do not introduce an exercise regimen without first consulting the doctor or physical therapist.

Entertainment

You may not only be responsible for meeting physical needs but additionally for meeting emotional needs. Part of this can be met by introducing some form of entertainment. Among possible options may be:

- encouraging more visiting by friends and family, whether other adult children, siblings, remote cousins or old friends,

- music; especially where there has been a lifelong interest in music

- reading (large print books are available for those with vision problems)

- television (especially for many elderly women the "soap operas" become a surrogate family; and "game" shows maintain a competitive interest)

- talk shows which discuss "human interest" topics

- crosswords

- hobbies that are still manageable

- crafts

- talking to grandchildren or old cronies about "the past"

- card games or other games such as monopoly

Whether we are sick or well, we do need peer company; peers act not only as someone to talk to but they can be confidants. Even as the caregiver needs to vent frustrations and perhaps discontent with the status quo, so do their bedbound or housebound care-recipients.

- encouraging more visiting by friends and family, whether other adult children, siblings, remote cousins or old friends,

- music; especially where there has been a lifelong interest in music

- reading (large print books are available for those with vision problems)

- television (especially for many elderly women the "soap operas" become a surrogate family; and "game" shows maintain a competitive interest)

- talk shows which discuss "human interest" topics

- crosswords

- hobbies that are still manageable

- crafts

- talking to grandchildren or old cronies about "the past"

- card games or other games such as monopoly

Whether we are sick or well, we do need peer company; peers act not only as someone to talk to but they can be confidants. Even as the caregiver needs to vent frustrations and perhaps discontent with the status quo, so do their bedbound or housebound care-recipients.

Sleeping

Proper rest is essential for us all. There are several needs that must be met to ensure that the person gets proper rest.

- The room should be comfortably either warm or cool, depending on the season.

- Enough pillows for comfort should be provided.

- Several layers of bed-clothes, instead of one very heavy layer, is usually more comfortable.

- The room should be comfortably darkened.

- A dim, but functional night-light may help if bathroom visits are necessary.

- Reading until sleep-time or soft radio talk or music shows can be soporific.

- Constipation, pain or leg cramps are among conditions which may affect sleep patterns. If there is a problem, consult the doctor.

Lifting

Improper lifting techniques may not only damage the caregiver's physical health, they will make the care-recipient feel insecure and may lead to injury.

- Ask the nurse or physical therapist to demonstrate proper lifting techniques. Learn the appropriate action to move the patient in the bed; from the bed to the chair; from the chair to a standing position; how to make the bed with her in it; how to get up and down stairs; in and out of a car — whichever lift is required.

- The handicapped person should be encouraged to participate in the lift to the extent that his residual abilities will allow.

Avoiding Pressure Sores

Pressure sores can cause untold misery to an already debilitated person. Therefore it is essential for every measure to be taken to prevent them from developing.

- Change his position in the bed at regular intervals (ask the nurse or doctor what they recommend).

- Keep the vulnerable areas clean and dry.

- Do not drag a patient in the bed as the skin may tear.

- Make sure the bed is crease-free and crumb-free.

- Be careful when either giving or removing a bedpan; always roll or lift the patient; never drag him.

- A water-cushion or water-bed may help someone who is practically immobile.

If pressure sores do develop, consult the doctor or nurse immediately. Follow any care-plan they recommend. Usually a nurse will monitor the bedsores and provide treatment.

"Progress, however,
of the best kind,
is comparatively slow.
Great results
cannot be achieved at once;
and we must be satisfies
to advance in life as we walk,
step by step."

Samuel Smiles

Adapting to New Living Arrangements

Some Question to Consider When Deciding

Whether a Parent Should Come to Live with You

The decision should not be made without first considering the important question — how the family interacts, the lay-out and location of your home and a realistic evaluation of how the arrangement is likely to function.

The Family's Evaluation

Everyone presently living in the household — you, your spouse, your children of whatever age and stage, anyone else presently living there and of course your parent, will have to adapt and make certain changes. Therefore it is important, as far as is feasible, for everyone to be part of the decision-making process and to voice any anxieties he or she may have.

In your evaluation, seriously ask whether your family is as stable as it should be — are there any serious health problems, family inculpabilities or other stressful situations. If problems already exist bringing another person into the household, however strong the bond between you, may put even more pressure on the family.

Another important question to ask is will the family cope if your parent becomes very frail or disabled and needs constant care and attention. Does the family depend on your income which would mean that you could not easily leave work to provide the needed care.

The first question then is that whether as a family, you feel that you can comfortably assimilate your parent into the household, and secondly, how it would cope long-term. Be realistic and frank in your assessment.

Your Parent's Evaluation

Your parent should also try to evaluate how she perceives the stability of your household, whether she believes she can indeed fit in and whether her being there may cause friction or stress. Of course, her decision will be influenced by other pressures that the family may not fully understand — among them her fear of becoming disabled and on her own, feeling she isn't coping well with the grieving process following the loss of her spouse, or being nervous in a big, empty house. These pressures may not enable her to be fully realistic about the long-term implications of such a move.

The following factors may help you make that decision.

A Closer Lokk at the Family's and Your Parent's Present Interaction Pattern and Pressures

- Historically what has your relationship been with your parent?

- Can you provide a close relationship—one in which she feels a definite part of the household and not just an appendage who is there because there didn't seem to be any other option?

- Is your spouse supportive and understanding about such an arrangement?

- Do your children get on with their grandparent?

- Has she interfered in the past?

- Are there any family differences or grievances smoldering which may come to the fore if you are living in the same household?

- Do you and your parent have any communication problems?

- Do you have different sets of values?

- If the children are still at home, do your views on child-rearing differ significantly?

- Do you enjoy being in one another's company?

- Who made the suggestion for your parent to come and live with you — did you make it, feeling it would be simpler than you making constant visits to see how she was getting on: was it made immediately after the funeral of your other parent; was it made on the spur of the moment, did she make you feel that you had no choice but to ask her to come, or was it after careful consideration?

- How much additional work will be involved in having her come to live with you; and who will do that work?

- Does your parent realize that in giving up her own home, she will be losing control over decisions she has been making for years/

- If the move is for financial reasons, how will she cope with feeling that you are taking her in?

- How much "quality time" will you and your spouse and children have to spend together, considering the demands that you already have on your time?

- Will she be made to feel an integral part of the family; joining in activities and decisions or will she be treated more as a guest?

- If she has her own part of the house, will her privacy be respected and will she respect your privacy?

- Would she be expected to do some of the household chores in return for being there?

- What arrangements will you make and how will you cope in the event that she needs constant care and attention?

- What is her attitude towards you getting services and professionals in to help look after her in the event that she needs care?

The Physical Attributes and Location of Your Home

- Will her bedroom and bathroom be on the same floor?

- Will she have her own bedroom and bathroom — in other words, reasonable privacy if she wants it?

- Will the whole family's living quarters become cramped by her moving in?

- Is the only accommodation you are able to offer, a small box room?

- How many of her things can she bring with her?

- Can you assimilate some of her "precious pieces" into your home?

- If your home safe for your parent?

- Is it easily adaptable if she becomes disabled, unable to use stairs, needs to use a cane, a walker or a wheelchair?

- Is the neighborhood safe?

- Would she have access to public transport?

- If there isn't transport close by and it she doesn't drive, would you be able to take her and fetch her when she goes out?

- Are there people in her age group near by?

- Would she have access to shops, theaters, galleries, etc. to help her pass the time?

The Financial Arrangements

- Would you expect her to pay her room and board?

- Would she be expected to make periodic financial gifts; how would household expenses in which she is immediately involved — food; light, etc. be divided up?

- Would any other family members help out financially?

- Of course any discussion should be handled as kindly and discreetly as possible, however real issues should be brought up. It is kinder in the end to uncover what might be real problems now, than to wait until she has moved in and find that the arrangement is causing stress to her and/or to the family.

Some Questions to Consider Before Moving Back to Live With Your Parent(s)

Such a decision should not be made on the spur of the moment. There is more than just a physical move involved. The following may help you to look at other options and consider the possible wide-ranging effects that moving back may have on your short-and long-term quality of life.

Firstly Other Possible Options

- Have you consulted your parent's physician about how adequately you parent can or cannot manage?

- Do you know what the long-term prognosis is?

- Have you investigated what services may fulfill his needs?

- Do you know for which of those services he may qualify for financial aid/

- Do you know how much he can afford to pay for services

- Have you considered holding a family conference and asking help from family members in meeting his needs; either by way of help or financial contributions toward bringing in outside help?

- Ask your employer whether you may have extra time beyond that now mandated, to sort out a caregiving support system that does not require you to return home.

You may well find that your parent can continue to be supported for longer in his own home without having to move back.

If not, then you may have no option but to move back and provide the quality of care he requires.

What are Some of the Possible Effect *On Your Life if* Moving Back Financially

- Short-term, if you have to give up work, you will almost certainly have to live on a reduced income.

- You may end up using up some portion of your reserves.

- Longer-term, your private and Social Security benefits will be affected.

- Your long-term career options may be seriously impeded; therefore impacting you longer-term earning potential.

Emotionally

- You will inevitably be relinquishing some of the independence you have achieved by living in separate accommodation.

- Your privacy may be seriously affected.

- Your care-recipient may begin to take your caring for granted.

- You may find yourself being treated as a "small child" again.

- You may find that gradually you lose your social contacts.

- You may become intra-dependent on the caregiving role.

- You may become resentful and frustrated and in turn, your mental health be affected.

Some Possible Coping Strategies

Accommodation-wise

- If financially feasible, keep your accommodation at least until you are sure you are happy with the arrangement or you are sure you have no other options.

To Preserve Your Health

- Try to introduce a caregiving schedule that gives you time to yourself.

- Get away for periodic breaks.

- Do your best to retain as much independence as you can.

- Introduce what supportive services you feel that you need, and are affordable.

Try to keep your care-recipient's other family and friends involved (this may not only alleviate the physical burden but the emotional one-to-oneness).

- Ask the Occupational Therapist what aids and equipment will give your care-recipient greater independence.

Moving back home is not an easy decision. Perhaps you may want to consult a social worker who can advise you about the steps you can take to meet the needs of your own particular situation.

Your goal should be to ensure that your parent receives the care she needs and that your own needs do not become subsumed in meeting those needs.

Later on, you will have to re-make your Life — if under pensionable age, you'll have to return to work and at

22. Adapting to New Living Arrangements

any age, you'll have to remake a social life for yourself. Therefore, you should take time over such a big decision, making sure you look at the possible short and long term impact.

Going Into a Nursing Home

It may be the most difficult decision you ever make. But at some point in the course of your loved one's Alzheimer's, you may find yourself face to face with the question: "Should we put him in a nursing home?"

We all grow up thinking that, when the time comes, we would never, ever put our parent, our spouse, or our siblings into a nursing home. And yet, life doesn't always oblige us. Reality forces us to consider the nursing home option, particularly when our loved one can no longer be watched all day long or when he needs specialized care. When conditions develop that are beyond our control or are potentially dangerous, family members must re-examine the appropriateness of in-home care. Health care professionals can help you evaluate and consider the options.

Here are some basic questions you should ask yourself.

- Can I continue to provide for the needs of our loved one at home on a 24-hour basis?

- Has the patient's health changed such that more nursing care and medical monitoring are required?

- Are my health concerns beginning to rival those of my loved one with Alzheimer's?

- Is the idea of a nursing home as unacceptable as it once was?

- Is in-home care contributing to the physical and emotional well-being of my loved one wearing me down?

- Could contact with my loved one improve with nursing home placement?

- Have physicians and other health care professionals recommended that my loved one go into a nursing home?

- Has caregiving in the home become ineffective in dealing with daily problems?

The more you can factor these considerations into your decision, the more likely you are to arrive at a decision satisfactory to all concerned. Of course, at this stage, your loved one may not to be able to contribute meaningfully to the decision.

As you consider where to place your loved one, start with the nursing homes in your area. In recent years, nursing homes have become much more aware of the needs of the Alzheimer's patient and the family. Many homes now have separate units, with specially trained staff to care for Alzheimer's patients. Some have special therapeutic programs for all family members.

To be certain that the home you choose gives care that meets your standards, look at as many homes as you are able. Compare them for price, as well as the ratio of patients to staff, the level of hygiene maintained, the cleanliness of rooms and hallways, safety features, the quality of the food — and all kinds of observations you can make by visiting the home and by talking to staff, residents, and families. You might also ask the home's administrators how much and what kinds of in-service education and training about Alzheimer's disease the staff are given. Perhaps as an added check, call your local chamber of commerce and your state's department of health to find out whether they seem merited.

Here are some of the points to weigh in making your choice.

- Is the facility a reasonable distance from your home? (Do not underestimate the importance of proximity to your home. If you are close enough to the nursing home, you will be more likely to visit more often.)

- Does the Alzheimer's unit have a special approach to caring for residents? (Beware of the unit that is just a way of grouping patients together rather than providing specialized services.)

- How familiar is the staff physician with Alzheimer's?

- How familiar are nursing, dietary, and activities staff with the special needs and problems of the Alzheimer's patient?

- How do staff members interact with Alzheimer's patients? (Try to catch them interacting without their knowledge of your presence. This will tell the real tale.)

- What kinds of activities are provided for the patients?

- What safety provisions have been made to keep patients from wandering or hurting themselves?

- Is there too much noise and confusion in the Alzheimer's unit? (Excessive noise might indicate that the unit is not being particularly well-managed.)

- How many nurses are on-duty at a given time? (Check this in the late evening hours as well — when some nursing homes are seriously understaffed.)

- Is there a safe area for the patients to walk or sit outside?

- Is the physical layout of the facility attractive, well-organized, and designed for the privacy needs of your loved one?

- What kinds of involvement does the facility offer the family? Are there support groups for family members to join? Are periodic conferences with family and the care team encouraged?

- How are medications and physical restraint devices used in behavior management? (If you see too many patients being restrained in their beds, or if it looks as though sedatives are too freely dispensed, there may be a problem. The laws governing the physical and chemical restraint of patients are detailed and strict. They include a provision that the home must get prior permission from the family. Certain forms of restraint are also illegal. No one can be restrained 24 hours a day.)

Once you've made the decision about which home your loved one should stay in, you will need to address some issues for yourself as well. These have to do with making the transition to having your relative cared for by "strangers." It is inevitable that you will feel some remorse that you are no longer able to care for your loved one; however, you should guard against letting the guilt get the upper hand. (When guilt gets in the way, the results can be disastrous: most relatives just stop coming to visit after awhile.)

Remind yourself of the strain and frustrations you've been experiencing. Give yourself permission to feel relieved that you no longer have a 24-hour-a-day caregiving job. Realize you can now visit your loved one more freely and with an open heart. Reaffirm to yourself that you have made a prudent, considered decision which, in the long run, will be best for everyone. You are taking care of your loved one — and yourselves — in the best way possible.

It is very important for the family carefully to make the transition from at-home care to active participation in nursing home care. For the patient, frequent, regular visits from family are critical. Your loved one may feel very disoriented in new surroundings, and your face and your voice will be familiar and reassuring.

Another reason for making frequent visits early on is that you can more effectively deal with adjustments that your loved one has to make. Close cooperation with the nursing home staff will ensure that your loved one receives the most appropriate care. By placing your loved one in a nursing home, you don't lose a relative — you "expand" your family of caregivers. If you can work with staff as you would with other family members, so much the better for everyone.

Communication between the patient's family and the nursing staff is the key. When the family is happy or unhappy with anything, they need to schedule a conference, just as they might do with their children's teachers. Staff should be open to discussing the care the patient is getting, and if there's anything at all they need to be doing differently.

A nursing home can look very sterile and cold to visitors. But it can be a nice, comfortable place to live, particularly once patients get used to predictable routines and non-threatening surroundings. Indeed, many Alzheimer's patients in the late stages of their illness often find more peace and comfort in a nursing home than in their own homes. In a good facility, their last months or years can be filled with comfort and relative happiness.

Nursing Home Selection

To Help You With Your Decision

What are Some Attributes to Look for in a Nursing Home? Vital several nursing homes ahead of time if you are going to need to transfer the responsibility for your loved one's care in the near future. Rate each home on a scale of 0 – 4.

(0 = unacceptable rating, 2 = average rating, 4 = excellent rating.)

Name of Institution

Among Questions to Consider	0	1	2	3	4
Is the structure clean, odor-free?					
Is it safe and secure?					
What is the ratio of trained to carry out their roles?					
Are staff adequately trained to carry out their roles?					
Are some staff specially trained to deal with those suffering from Alzheimer's disease?					

Are staff licensed?					
Is the facility licensed?					
What is the accommodation like?					
Do patients have extra pillows, blankets, etc.?					
What bathing facilities are there?					
What intensive care is provided?					
What procedures are used to prevent bed-bound patients from developing bedsores?					
What procedures are used in the event the patient cannot feed himself?					
What is the scope of the activities program? Are meals well-balanced? (Look at menus.) Do staff appear to be sensitive to patient's needs? (Discreetly talk to patients and their families.)					
What therapies are provided?					
Is there a general exercise program, based on patient's abilities to participate?					
What is the complaints procedure?					

Are the charges all inclusive; which services are extra?					
How much can you get involved; walking, feeding visiting?					
Are visiting hours flexible, open, definite?					
What spiritual guidance is there — does a chaplain visit regularly; are there church services?					
Do the patients look contented, agitated, anxious, unhappy?					
What is the staff hierarchy?					

Meditation

"If a person's basic state of mind is serene and calm then it is possible for this inner peace to overwhelm a painful physical experience. On the other hand, if someone is suffering from depression, anxiety, or any form of emotional distress, then even if he or she happens to be enjoying physical comforts, he will not really be able to experience the happiness that these could bring."

John Quincy Adams

Hot Lines

A

Adoption
National Council for Adoption   800-862-3678

Aging
Administration of Aging/Department
of Health and human Services   202-401-4634
Central Massachusetts Agency on Aging   800-244-3032
Eldercare Locator   800-677-1116
National Institute on Aging   800-677-1116
National Council of the Aging, Inc.   800-677-1116
Older Women's League   202-567-2606

AIDS
AIDS info (http://aidsinfo.nih.gov)   800-448-0440
AIDS Clinical Trials Information Service   800-874-2572
Committee of Ten Thousand (AIDS)   800-488-2688
National AIDS Clearinghouse   800-458-5231
            TTY/TDD   800-243-1098
National AIDS Hotline   800-342-2437
National Indian AIDS Hotline   800-283-6880
Project Inform   800-822-7422
Treatment Information Services   800-448-044
            TDD   800-480-3739

Alzheimer's Disease
Alzheimer's Association   800-272-3900
Alzheimer's Disease Education and
Referral Center   800-438-4380
Alzheimer's Foundation of America   866-232-8484
French Foundation for
Alzheimer Research   310-445-4650
National Caregiving Foundation   800-222-5864

Arthritis
Arthritis Foundation Information Line   800-283-7800

Assisting Living
Assisted Living Federation of America   703-691-8100
Eldercare Locator   800-677-1116

Autism
Autism Society of America   800-328-8476

B

Back Injury, Prevention of American
Academy of Orthopedic Surgeons   847-823-7186

Batten Disease
Batten Disease Support and Research
Association   800-448-4570

Blind
American Council for the Blind   800-424-8666
American Foundation for the Blind, Inc.   800-232-5463
Guide Dog Foundation for the Blind   800-548-4337
Lighthouse Center for Vision and Agin   800-334-4597
National Association for Parents of the
Visually Impaired   800-562-6265
National Center for Sight   800-221-3004
National Eye Research Foundation   847-564-4652
Prevent Blindness America   800-331-2020

Brain Tumor
American Brain Tumor Association   800-886-2282
Children's Brain Tumor Foundation   866-228-4673
National Brain Tumor Society   617-924-9997

Breastfeeding
La Leche League International   800-227-2345

C

Cancer

American Cancer Society Cancer Response Line	800-227-2345
American Institute for Cancer Research	800-843-8114
Cancer Care Inc.	800-813-4673
Cancer Help Line	800-862-2215
Cancer Hope Network	877-467-3638
Cancer Information Service	800-422-6237
Candlelighters Childhood Cancer Foundation	503-235-5722
Chemocare (Cancer)	800-552-4366
National Cancer Institute (Cancer Information Service)	800-422-6237
National Children's Cancer Society	800-532-6459
Y-Me National Organization for Breast Cancer Information and Support	800-221-2141

Caregiving

Family Caregivers Alliance	800-445-8106
National Caregiving Foundation	800-930-1357

Care Managers

National Association of Professional Geriatric Care Managers	520-881-8008

Cerebral Palsy

United Cerebral Palsy Association, Inc.	800-872-5827

Children

Boys & Girls Hotline	800-448-3000
Cancer Hope Network	877-467-3638
Cystic Fibrosis Foundation	800-344-4823
Fathers Flanagan's Boys Town	800-448-3000

Federation for Children with Special Needs	800-331-0688
Human Growth Foundation (Growth Disorders in Children)	800-451-6434
National Center for Missing and Exploited Children	800-843-5678
National Children's Cancer Society	800-532-6459
National Clearinghouse on Child Abuse and Neglect Information	800-394-3366
National Easter Seals Society	800-221-6827
National Information Center for Children and Youth with Disabilities	800-695-0285
Safe Sitter	800-255-4089
Shriner's Hospital Referral Line	800-237-5055
Sturge-Weber Disease Foundation	800-627-5482
Sudden Infant Death Syndrome	800-221-7437
Virginia Missing Children Information Clearinghouse	800-822-4453

Craniofacial Handicaps

American Cleft Palate-Craniofacial Association	800-242-5338
Children's Craniofacial Association	800-535-3643
Faces National Association for the Craniofacial Handicapped	800-332-2373
National Foundation for Facial Reconstruction (My Face)	212-263-6656

Crohn's Disease

Crohn's and Colitis Foundation of America	800-932-2423

D

Deafness

Cochlear Implant Information Center	800-458-4999

Voice/TTY	800-523-5798
Deaf, Hard of Hearing and Speech Disabled	800-877-8339
Hear Now	800-648-HEAR
National Institute on Deafness and Other Communication Disorders Information Clearinghouse	800-241-1044
Starkey Foundation	800-328-8602

Depression

| National Institute of Mental Health | 800-421-4211 |

Diabetes

American Diabetes Association	800-342-2383
American Diabetes Foundation	800-232-3472
Diabetes Information Clearinghouse	800-860-8747
National Diabetes Outreach Program	800-438-5383

Domestic Violence

| National Domestic Violence Hotline | 800-799-7233 |

Down Syndrome

| National Down Syndrome Congress | 800-232-6372 |
| National Down Syndrome Society Hotline | 800-221-640 |

Drugs/Medicines

Alternative Medicine	888-644-6226
Department of Health and Human Services	877-696-6775
Drug Prevention and Treatment	800-662-4357
Drug Treatment Referrals	800-662-4357
Pharmaceutical Research and Manufacturers of America	800-762-4636

(Directory of pharmaceutical companies that provide medicines to physicians whose patients cannot afford them.)

Dwarfism
Little People of America   888-LPA-2001

Dyslexia
Dyslexia Society International   800-222-3123
National Dyslexia Research Foundation   946-642-7303
The Dyslexia Foundation   941-807-0499

Dystonia
Dystonia Foundation   800-377-3978
National Spasmodic Dysphonia
Association   800-795-6732

E

Education
Federal Student Aid Information Center   800-433-3243
Student Financial Aid program
information   800-730-8913

Eldercare
Eldercare Locator   800-677-1116

Elimination Tract Diseases
National Foundation for Ileitis & Colitis   800-343-3637

Emergency Air Transportation
Care Flight Air Critical Care   800-282-6878

Epilepsy
Citizens United for Research in Epilepsy   312-255-1801
Epilepsy Foundation of America   800-332-1000

Equipment and Products
Abledata, National Rehabilitation Center 800-227-0216
800-346-2742

G

Gastrointestinal Disorders
International Foundation for Functional
Gastrointestinal Disorders   212-249-5402

Grief Recovery
Grief Recovery Institute   818-907-9600

H

Head
Migraine Research Foundation/Migraine
& Pain Fund   212-249-5402
National Brain Injury Foundation
Family Hotline   800-444-6443
National Headache Foundation   800-843-2256

Health
Health Care Information Clearinghouse   800-358-9295
Health Practitioner Helpline   800-767-6732
National Health Information Center   800-336-4797
National Institute of Health
(Clinical Studies)   800-411-1222

Heart
American Heart Association   800-242-8721

Helping Aids
Eldercare Locator   800-677-1116
Keiser Corporation
(Step in the Right Direction)   800-888-7009
Lifeline (Personal Response &
Support Services)   800-451-0525

NU STEP (Fitness)	800-322-2209
Oreck Corporation (Housekeeping)	800-535-8810
Philips Lfeline (Emergency Call System)	800-548-8805
Physician Problems (Local Solutions)	
General Medicine	800-979-9595
Protect Alert Emergency	
Response Systems, Inc.	800-862-1288
Smart Caregivers Corporation	
(Housekeeping)	800-650-3637

Herpes
| American Social Health Association | 800-230-6039 |

High Blood Cholesterol
| National Heart, Lung and Blood Institute | 800-575-9355 |

High Blood Pressure
| National Heart, Lung and Blood Institute | 800-575-9355 |

Hospice
| Children's Hospice International | 703-837-1500 |
| Hospice Education Institute Hospicelink | 800-331-1620 |

Hospitality Houses
| National Association of Hospitality Houses, Inc. | 800-542-9730 |

Huntington's Disease
| Heredity Disease Foundation | 212-928-2121 |

Immunization
| Immunization Referral Locator Service | 800-232-4636 |

Incontinence
| Help for Incontinent People | 800-252-3337 |

Simon Foundation for Continence   800-237-4666

Insurance
Life Rates of America   800-457-2837
Medicaid   800-633-4227
Medicare   800-633-4227
National Insurance Consumer Helpline   800-942-4224
Veterans Administration   800-827-1000

K

Kidney
American Association of Kidney Patients   800-749-2257
American Kidney Fund   800-638-8299
Kidney and Urologic Disease Information   800-891-5390
National Kidney Foundation   800-622-9010
Polycystic Kidney Disease Research
Foundation   800-753-2873

L

Lead Poisoning
National Lead Information Center   800-424-5323

Leukemia
Leukemia Society of America   800-955-4572

Liver
American Lung Association   800-586-4872

Lupus
Lupus Foundation of America   800-558-0121

Lymphedema
National Lymphedema Network   800-541-3259

M

Medic Alert
Medic Alert Foundation   800-432-5378

Medicare
Medicare Telephone Hotline   800-633-4227

Mental Health
The Arc of the United States   800-433-5255
Mental health Information Clearinghous 800-400-2742
National Depressive and Manic
Depressive Association   800-826-3632
National Institute of Mental Health   800-421-4211
National Mental Health Association   800-969-6642
National Mental Health Consumers'
Self-Help Clearinghouse   800-553-4539
Panic Disorder Education Program —
National Institute of Mental Health   800-647-2642

Multiple Sclerosis
Multiple Sclerosis Association of America 800-532-7667
MS Friends   866-673-7436
Multiple Sclerosis Foundation   800-225-6495
National Multiple Sclerosis Society   800-344-4867

Muscular Dystrophy
Muscular Dystrophy Association   800-344-4863

Myasthenia Gravis
Myasthenia Gravis Foundation of America 800-541-5454

N

Neurofibromatosis
Children's Tumor Foundation   800-323-7938

Neurological Disorders
American Academy of Neurology
Foundation   800—879-1960
American Spasmodic Torticollis
Association   800-487-8385

Amyotrophic Lateral Sclerosis
Association   800-782-4747
National Institute of Neurological
Disorders and Stroke   800-352-9424

Neuromuscular Diseases
ALS Association   800-782-4747
Moebius Syndrome Foundation   660-834-3406
Muscular Dystrophy Association   800-344-4863
Neuropathy Association   212-692-0662

O

Obsessive-Compulsive Disorder
Obsessive-Compulsive Foundation   617-973-5801

Organ Donations
The Living Bank   800-528-2971
Organ Transplant Fund, Inc.   800-489-3863

P

Pain
Neuropathy Association   212-692-0662

Panic Disorder
National Institute of Mental Health   800-617-2612

Paralysis
Christopher Reeves Paralysis Foundation 800-225-0292
National Spinal Cord Injury Association 800-962-9629

Parkinson's Disease
American Parkinson's Disease Association 800-223-2732
International Essential Tremor Foundation 888-387-3667
Michael J. Fox Foundation for
Parkinson's Research   800-708-7644
National Ataxia Foundation   763-553-0020
National Parkinsons Foundation   800-327-4545

Florida Residents	800-433-7022
Parkinson's Disease Foundation	800-457-6676
Society for Progressive Supranuclear Palsy	800-457-4777

R

Rare Diseases

Aplastic Anemia Foundation of America	800-747-2820
Charcot-Marie-Tooth Association	800-606-2682
Cornelia De Lange Syndrome Foundation	800-223-8355
FHistiocytosis-X Association of America	800-548-2758
National Fragile X Foundation	800-688-8765
National Sjogren's Syndrome Association	800-475-6473
National Tuberous Sclerosis Association	800-225-6872
Tourette Syndrome Association	800-237-0717
Turner's Syndrome Society	800-365-9944
United Scleroderma Association	800-722-4673

Recreation

| American Therapeutic Recreation Association | 601-450-2872 |
| National Therapeutic Recreation Society | 703-858-0784 |

Rehabilitation

| National Rehabilitation Center | 800-346-2742 |

Reye's Syndrome

| National Reye's Syndrome Foundation | 800-233-7393 |

S

Sickle Cell Disease

| Sickle Cell Disease Association of America | 800-421-8456 |

Sight Impairment

| Braille Institute | 800-272-4553 |

Skin Problems

First-Foundation for Ichthyosis and Related Skin Types, Inc.	800-545-3286
National Organization for Albinism and Hypopigmentation	800-473-2310
National Psoriasis Foundation	800-248-0886

Social Security

Social Security Administration	800-772-1213
TTD	800-325-0778

Spinal Cord

Ankylosing Spondylitis Association	800-777-8189
Families Spinal Muscular Atrophy	800-886-1762
Spinal Bifida Association of America	800-621-3141
United Leukodystrophy Foundation	800-728-5483

Stress

American Institute of Stress	914-963-1200

Stroke

American Stroke Association	888-478-7653
Brain Attack Coalition	301-496-5751
National Institute of Neurological & Stroke Disorders	800-352-9424
National Stroke Association	800-787-6537
Stroke Connection Network	800-553-6321

Stuttering

National Center for Shuttering	800-221-2483

Substance Abuse

Al-Anon Family Group Headquarters	800-356-9996
National Clearinghouse for Alcohol and Drug Information	800-729-6686
National Drug Information Treatment and Referral Hotline	800-662-4357

Suicide
VA Suicide Hotline   800-723-TALK

Support Groups
Alliance of Genetic Support Groups   800-336-4363
Community Transportation Association
of America   800-527-8279
FCC Disability Rights   888-225-5322
Hospice Foundation of America   800-854-3402
Medicare Hotline   800-633-4227
National Hospice and Palliative Care   800-658-8898
Parents Without Partners   800-637-7974
Well Spouse Foundation   800-838-0879

T

Thyroid
Myasthenia Gravis Foundation   800-541-5454

Transplant
National Bone Marrow Transplant
Program   -627-7890

Trauma
American Trauma Society   800-556-7890
Brain Injury Association of America   800-444-6443
Brain Trauma Foundation   212-772-0608

Tumor
American Brain Tumor Association   800-886-2282

V

Vestibular Disorders
Vestibular Disorders Association   800-837-8428

Veterans
VA Benefits   800-827-1000

Education (GI Bill)	888-442-4551
VA Health Care Benefits	877-222-8387

Web Sites

Alphabetical Listing

A

A

American Heart Association...........www.americanheart.og
American Academy of Neurology....https://www.aan.com/
Assisted Living..........................http://www.eldercare.gov

Amputee
Amputee Coalition of America......http://www.amputee-coalition.org/

Assistive Technology
Active Forever...............................www.activeforever.com
Dynamic Living.........................www.dynamic-living.com

B

Blind
AbilityOne Program.............https://www.abilityone.org/
America Foundation for the Blind...............www.afb.org

Books
Project Gutenberg (free online books)...............http://www.gutenberg.org/
Overdrive (download library materials-free)......www.overdrive.com

Brain Injury
Brain Injury Association of Michigan.......http://www.biami.org/
Brain Injury Association of America.....http://www.biaisa.org/
Brain Injury Resource Center.....http://headinjury.com/
Brain Trauma Foundation.......https://www.braintrauma.org/

National Inst, Neurological
Disorders & Stroke…................http://www.ninds.nih.
gov/
North American Brain
Injury Society……....…………..…http://www.nabis.
rog/
Traumatic Brain
Injury.Com…….......http://www.traumaticbraininjury.
com/
Traumatic Brain Injury
Survival Guide……….....…........http://www.tbguide.
com

Brain Tumor

American Brain Tumor Association…http://www.abta.
org/
National Brain Tumor
Society…..................................http://www.braintumor.
org/

C

Caregiver

Care for the Caregiver...…………....aarp.org/caregiving
National Caregiver
Foundation....................http://caregivingfoundationorg/
National Famil Caregivers Association.............www.
nfcacares.org

Cooking

The Cooking
Channe…..…http://www.cookingchanneltv.com/home.
html

D

Disability

Disability Information and
Resources..................................http://www.makoa.org/

E

Education
Free online classes and
tutorials............................http://www.gcflearnfree.org/

Employment
Job Accommodation Network...........http://askjan.org/

Entertainment
Project Gutenberg
(free online books)..................ttp://www.gutenberg.oeg/

F

Facebook...................................www.facebook.com

H

Health
Government on
Health................http://nccam.nih.gov/health/atoz.htm
Lucinia Health...............http://lusciniahealth.com/
Network of Care.....................www.networkofcare.org
Web MD....................................www.webmd.com

L

LIBRARY
Public Libraries.........http://www.publiclibraries.com/

M

Medical Equipment
Active Forever.............................www.activeforever.com

Dynamic Living......................www.dynamic-living.com

Medical Information

United States National Library
of Medicine.............................http://www.nlm.nih.gov/
Medicare..............................http://www.medicare.gov/

Meditation Music

Live 365.com....http://www.live365.com/new/index.live

Meditation Video

Gift of Inner Peace...........................www.giftofpeace.org
Mayo Clinic....www.mayoclinic.com/health/meditation/
MM00623

Meditation Techniques

Meditation
Techniques...www.ananda.org/meditation/technique.
html-
Meditation Society…...........www.meditationsociety.com

Movies

Overdrive (download library
materials-free)...................................www.overdrive.com
Hulu...http://www.hulu.com/
Live 365.com...http://www.live365.com/new/index.live
Solo Piano.....................................…www.solopiano.com
Soundclick.........................http://www.soundclick.com/

N

National Stroke Associations…http://www.stroke.org/
site/PageNavigator/HOME
National Headache
Foundation..........................http://www.headaches.org/

O

Online Social Pages

Facebook...www.facebook.com

Myspace..www.myspace.com

P

Pain
American Pain Foundation....http://painfoundation.org/
American Chronic Pain Association...http://theacpa.org/

Paralysis
Paralysis Research Center……...........www.paralysis.org
Spinal Cord Injury……........http://www.spinalcord.org/
Spinal Cord Injury Information
Pages……......................http://www.sci-info-pages.com/

Poison
American Association of Poison Control
Centers…...................................…http://www.aapcc.org/

Prescription Assistance
Copay Relief...www.copays.org
Needy Meds....................................www.needymeds.org
Partnership for Prescription Assistanc.......www.parx.org

R

Reading
National Sleep Foundation...http://sleepfoundation.org/

Social Security
Social Security………………...............…..http://ssa.gov/

Spinal Cord Injury
National Spinal Cord Injury
Association…....................................www.spinalcord.org
Spinal Cord Injury Information
Pages……...................................www.sci-info-pages.com

Sports

Disabled Sports USA..…http://disabledsportsusa.org/
Wintergreen Adaptive
Sports…..............http://wintergreenadaptivesports.org/

Stroke

American Stroke Association..http://strokeassociation.
org/STROKEORG/
Brain Attack Coalition..........http://www.stroke-site.org/
National Institute of Neurological Disorders &
Stroke…...www.ninds.nih.gov

Suicide

National Suicide
Prevention..................www.suicidepreventionlifeline.org

V

Veteran

U.S. Department of Veteran Affairs............http://va.gov/

W

Wellness Web MD...................http://www.webmd.com/

Emergency Procedures

Keep this information up to date.

Care-Recipient

Name _____

Nickname _____

Address _____

Phone Number _____

Date of Birth _____

Social Security # _____

Disease/illness/condition _____

Blood Type _____

Organ donation status _____

Other _____

_____

_____

_____

Caregiver

Address _____

Home phone _____ Work phone _____

Other _____

_____

_____

Emergency Phone Numbers Other Than 911

Police _____

Fire_____

Ambulance _____

Hospital _____

Other _____

_____

_____

In case of illness or accident, contact

Doctor(s)

Name_____

Adress_____

Office phone_____Home Phone_____

Name_____

Adress_____

Office phone_____Home phone_____

Spouse, Significant Other, Relative, Friend, or Neighbor

Name_____

Office phone_____Home phone_____

Address_____

Name_____

Office phone_____Home phone_____

Address_____

Pharmacy

Name_____

Address_____

Phone Number_____

Hours_____

Medication(s)_____

_____

Medication producing allergic reaction_____

_____

Allergies_____

Special instruction_____

_____

Health Insurance Company

Name_____

Policy number_____

Phone number_____

Medicare ID number_____

Emergency Procedures

Legal and Financial

Name_____

Address_____

Phone Number_____

Tax Consultant/Accountant

Name_____

Address_____

Phone number_____

Banker

Name_____

Address_____

Phone number_____

Insurance Agent

Name_____

Address_____

Phone number_____

Other

_____

_____

_____

_____

Church/Synagogue/Temple/Mosque

Name_____

Phone_____

Priest, pastor or rabbi_____

Funeral Arrangements

_____

_____

_____

The following Information concerns the care-recipient's ability to perform activities of daily living.

	Yes	No
Dressing	—	—
Undressing	—	—
Bathing	—	—
Toileting	—	—
Dentures	—	—
Eyeglasses	—	—
Hearing aid	—	—
Other		

_____

_____

The following information concerns any special handling and established routines of the care-recipient.

Strange behaviors _____
_____
_____

Special Skills _____
_____
_____

Favorite Activities _____
_____
_____

Things that may agitate _____
_____
_____

Food intolerance _____
_____
_____

Special dietary needs _____
_____
_____

Emergency Procedures

Meal times

Breafast_____

Lunch_____

Dinner_____

Favorite foods

Meats_____

_____

_____

Vegetables_____

_____

_____

Fruits_____

_____

_____

Desserts_____

_____

_____

Beverages_____

_____

_____

Favorite snacks_____

_____

_____

Bath time_____

_____

_____

Bedtime_____

Awakens in A.M. at_____

Notes

_____

_____

_____

_____

_____

_____

_____

_____

_____

_____

_____

_____

_____

_____

_____

_____

_____

_____

_____

_____

_____

Health Care Planning

Using Advance Directives

Optional Advance Directives
Your Forms Included

Adults can decide for themselves whether they want medical treatment. This right to decide — to say yes or no to proposed treatment — applies to treatments that extend life, like a breathing machine or a feeding tube. Tragically, accident or illness can take away a person's ability to make health care decisions. But decisions still have to be made. If you cannot do so, someone else will. These decisions should reflect your own values and priorities.

You can do health care planning, through "advance directives." An advance directive can be used to name a health care agent. This is someone you trust to make health care decisions for you. An advance directive can also be used to say what your treatment preferences are, especially about treatments that might be used to sustain your life.

There are two optional forms on the following pages. The shorter one is titled "Living Will." The longer one is titled "Advance Directive," and it has two parts, Part A and Part B. This pamphlet will explain how to use them. These forms are intended to be guides. You may complete all of form, or only the parts you want to use. You are not required by law to use these forms. Different forms, written the way you want, may also be used.

These optional forms can be filled out without going to a lawyer. But if there is anything you do not understand, you might want to talk with a lawyer. You can also ask your doctor to explain the medical issues. You should tell your doctor that you made an advance directive and give your doctor a copy.

You need two witnesses to your signature on these forms. Nearly any adult can be a witness. If you name a health care agent, though, that person may not be a witness. Also, one of the witnesses must be a person who would not financially benefit by your death or handle your estate. You do not need to have the form notarized.

Once you make an advance directive, it remains in effect unless you revoke it. It does not expire. You should review what you've done occasionally. Things might change in your life, or your attitudes might change. You are free to amend or revoke an advance directive at any time. Tell your doctor and anymore else who has a copy of your advance directive if you amend it or revoke it.

Health Care Agents

You can name anyone you want (except, in general, someone who works for a health care facility where you are receiving care) to be your health care agent. To name a health care agent, use Part A of the advance directive form. Your agent will speak for you and make decisions based on what you would want done or your best interests. You decide how much power your agent will have to make health care decisions. You can also decide when you want your agent to have this power – right away, or only after your doctors agree that you are not able to decide for yourself.

You can pick a family member as a health care agent, but you don't have to. Remember that your agent will have the power to make important treatment decisions, even if other people close to you might urge a different decision.

Choose the person best qualified to be your health care agent. Also, consider picking a back-up agent, in case your first choice isn't available when needed. Don't pick someone without telling the person. Make sure that the person you pick understands what's most important to you. When the time comes for decisions, your health care agent should do what you would want.

The forms included with this *Caregiver's Support Kit* ® do not give anyone power to handle your money. There isn't a standard form we can send. Talk to your lawyer about planning for financial issues in case of incapacity.

Health Care Instructions

You also have the right to use an advance directive to say what you want about future treatment issues. If you name a health care agent and make decisions about treatment in an advance directive, your agent will be bound by whatever decisions you make unless you say otherwise.

If you want, you can make a limited kind of advance directive called a living will. A living will lets you decide about life-sustaining procedures in two situations: death from a terminal condition is imminent despite the application of life sustaining procedures, and a condition of permanent unconsciousness called a persistent vegetative state.

You also have the right to give broader health care instructions by using Part B of the longer form. Part B of the advance directive lets you decide about life-sustaining procedures in three situations: terminal condition, persistent vegetative state, and end-stage condition. An end-stage condition is an advanced, progressive, and incurable condition resulting in complete physical dependency. One example is advanced

Alzheimer's disease. You can also use Part B of the advance directive to make health care decisions in addition to those dealing with life sustaining procedures. If you fill out Part B, you should not fill out the living will form too.

Both the living will form and Part B let you decide separately, if you want, about artificially supplied nutrition and hydration, often called "tube feeding." Also, women who fill out either form can say whether pregnancy is to have any effect on their treatment decisions.

Did You Remember To ...

☐ Fill out, sign, and have witnessed Part A of the advance directive if you want to name a health care agent?

☐ Name a back-up agent in case your first choice as health care agent is not available when needed?

☐ Talk to your agent and back-up agent about your values and priorities, and decide whether that's enough guidance or whether you also want to make specific health care decisions that your agent must follow?

☐ Fill out (choosing carefully among alternatives), sign, and have witnessed either a living will or the broader Part B of the advance directive, but only if you want to make specific decisions?

☐ Make sure your health care agent (if you named one), you family, and your doctor know about your advance care planning?

☐ Give a copy of your advance directive to your health care agent, family members, doctor, and hospital or nursing home if you are a patient there?

For additional copies of this, please contact:

The National Caregiving Foundation

P.O. Box 1176

Dunkirk, MD 20754

Frequently Asked Questions About Advance Directives

1. Must I use any particular form?

No. Optional forms are provided, but you may change them or use different forms altogether. Of course, no health care provider may deny you care simply because you decided not to fill out a form

2. Who can be picked as a health care agent?

Anyone who is 18 or older except, in general, an owner, operator, or employee of a health care facility where a patient is receiving care.

3. Who can witness an advance directive?

Two witnesses are needed. Generally, any competent adult can be a witness, including your doctor or other health care provider (but be aware that some facilities have a policy against their employees serving a witnesses). If you name a health care agent, that person cannot be a witness for any of your advance directives. Also, one of the two witnesses must be someone who (i) will not receive money or property from your estate and (ii) who is not the one you have named to handle your estate after your death.

4. Do the forms have to be notarized?

No, but if you travel frequently to another state, check with a knowledgeable lawyer to see if that state requires notarization.

5. Do any of these documents deal with financial matters?

No. If you want to plan for financial matters, talk with your lawyer.

6. When using these forms to make a decision, how do I show the choices that I have made?

Write your initials next to the statement that says what you want. Don't use checkmarks or Xs. Then draw lines all the way through other statements that do not say what you want. Please don't make inconsistent choices. For example, if you initial any or all of items 1,2, and 3 on Part B of the advance directive, do not initial item 5. Draw lines through it instead. Also, be very careful about item 4. Draw lines through it if you want to make sure that you get pain relief medication.

7. Should I fill out both the living will form and the advance directive form?

It depends on what you want to do. If all you want to do is name a health care agent, just fill out Part A of the advance directive. If you want to give treatment instructions, fill out either the living will form or Part B of the advance directive (not both). The living will form lets you decide about life-sustaining procedures in the event of terminal condition or persistent vegetative state but also "end-stage condition." Part B also lets you make health care decisions that deal with situations other than life-sustaining procedures. Be aware that, if you name a health care agent and

give treatment instructions, the agent will be bound
by your decisions unless you say otherwise.

8. Are these forms valid in another state?

It depends on the law of the other state. Most states
will honor an advance directive made somewhere else.

**9. To whom should I give copies of my advance
directive?**

Give copies to your doctor, your health care agent if
you name one; hospital or nursing home if you will
be staying there, and family members or friends who
should know of your wishes.

**10. Does the federal law on medical records privacy
(HIPAA) require special language about my health
care agent?**

Under HIPAA, a health care agent is a "personal
representative" who can get access to your medical
records. In Part A of the advance directive, at the
beginning of item 2A, you might want to write in
these words: "As my personal representative,

**11. If I have an advance directive, do I also need an
Emergency Medical Services Palliative Care/Do Not
Resuscitate Order?**

Yes. If you don't want ambulance personnel to try to
resuscitate you in the event of cardiac or respiratory
arrest, you mush have an EMS Palliative Care/DNR
Order signed by your private physician.

**12. Does the EMS Palliative Care/DNR Order have to
be in a particular form?**

Yes. Ambulance personnel have very little time to
evaluate the situation and act appropriately. Therefore,
it is not practical to ask them to interpret documents

that may vary in form and content. Instead, a standardized order form has been developed.

13. Can I use an advance directive to make an organ donation?

Yes. A special form for that purpose is included.

If you have other questions, please talk to your doctor or your lawyer.

Living Will

(Optional Form)

If I am not able to make an informed decision regarding my health care, I direct my health care provides to follow my instructions as set forth below. *(Initial those statements you wish to be included in the document and cross through those statements, which do not apply.)*

A. If my death from a terminal condition id=s imminent and even if life-sustaining procedures are used there is no reasonable expectation of my recovery:

_____ I direct that my life not be extended by life-sustaining procedures, including the administration of nutrition and hydration artificially.

_____ I direct that my life not be extended by life-sustaining procedures, except that if I am unable to take food by mouth, I wish to receive nutrition and hydration artificially.

_____ I direct that, even in a terminal condition, I be given all available medical treatment in accordance with acceptable health care standards.

b. If I am in a persistent vegetative state, that is, if I am not conscious and am not aware of my environment nor able to interacts with others, and there is no reasonable expectation of my recovery.

_____ I direct that my life not be extended by life-sustaining procedures, expect that if I am unable to take food by mouth, I wish to receive nutrition and hydration artificially.

_____ I direct that, even a terminal condition, I be given all available medical treatment in accordance with acceptable health care standards.

C. If I am pregnant, my decision concerning life-sustaining procedures shall be modified as follows:

_____

_____

_____

_____

_____

Living Will (continued)

By signing below, I indicate that I am emotionally and mentally competent to make this Living Will and that I understand its purpose and effect.

_____   _____
(Date)   (Signature of Declarant)

The declarant signed or acknowledged signing this Living Will in my presence and, based upon my personal observation, the declarant appears to be a competent individual.

_____   _____
(Witness)   (Witness)

_____   _____

_____   _____

_____   _____

_____   _____
(Signatures and Addresses of Two Witnesses)

Advance Directive

Part A

Appointment of Health Care Agent

(Optional Form)

(Cross through this whole part of the form if you do not want to appoint a health care agent to make health care decisions for you. If you do want appoint an agent, cross through any times in the form that you do not want to apply.)

I, _____,

residing at_____

_____

Appoint the following individual as my agent to make health care decisions for me: _____

_____

_____

_____

(Full Name, Address, and Telephone Number of Agent)

Optional: If this agent is unavailable or is unable or unwilling to act as my agent, then I appoint the following person to act in this capacity:

_____

_____

_____

(Full Name, Address, and Telephone Number of Back-up Agent)

Advance Directive Part A (continued)

My agent has full power and authority to make health care decisions for me, including the power of:

1. Request, receive, and review any information, oral or written, regarding my physical or mental health, including, but not limited to, medical care facility; and

2. Consent to the provision, withholding, or withdrawal of health care, including, inappropriate circumstances, life sustaining procedures.

3. The authority of my agent is subject to the following provisions and limitations:

4. If I am pregnant, may agent shall follow these specific instructions:

5. My agent's authority becomes operative *(initial only the one option that applies):*

   When my attending physician and a second physician determine that I am incapable of making an informed decision regarding my health care; or When this document is signed.

6. My agent is to make health care decisions for me based on the health care instructions I give in this document and on my wishes as otherwise known to my agent. If my wishes are unknown or unclear, my agent is to make health care decisions for me in accordance with, my best interest, to be determined by my agent after considering the benefits, burdens,

and risks that might result from a given treatment or course of treatment, or from the withholding or withdrawal of a treatment or course of treatment.

7. My agent shall not be liable for the costs of care based solely on this authorization.

By signing below, I indicate that I am emotionally and mentally competent to make this appointment of a health care agent and that I understand its purpose and effect.

_____   _____
(Date)   (Signature of Declarant)

The declarant signed or acknowledged signing this appointment of a health care agent in my presence and, based upon my personal observation, the declarant appears to be a competent individual.

_____   _____
(Witness)   (Witness)

_____   _____
_____   _____
_____   _____

(Signature and Address of Two Witnesses)

Advance Directive

Part B

Health Care Instructions
(Optional Form)

*(Cross through this whole part of the form if you do not want to use it to give health care instructions. If you do want to complete this portion of the form, **initial** those statements you want to be included in the document and cross through those statements that do not apply.)*

If I am incapable of making an informed decision regarding my health care, I direct my health care providers to follow my instructions as set forth below. (**Initial** all those that apply.)

1. If my death from a terminal condition is imminent and even if life-sustaining procedures are used there is no reasonable expectation of my recovery:

   _____ I direct that my life not be extended by life-sustaining procedures, including the administration of nutrition and hydration of my recovery:

   _____ I direct that my life not be extended by life-sustaining procedures, except that if I am unable to take food by mouth, I wish to receive nutrition and hydration artificially.

2. If I am in a persistent vegetative state, that is, if I am not conscious and am not aware of my environment nor able to interact with others, and there is no reasonable expectation of my recovery:

_____ I direct that my life not be extended by life-sustaining procedures, including the administration of nutrition and hydration artificially.

_____ I direct that my life not be extended by life-sustaining procedures, except that if I am unable to take food by mouth, I wish to receive nutrition and hydration artificially.

3. If I have an end-stage condition, that is, a condition caused by injury, disease, or illness, as a result pf which I have suffered severe and permanent deterioration indicated by incompetency and complete physical dependency and for which, to a reasonable degree of medical certainty, treatment of the irreversible condition would be medically ineffective:

_____ I direct that my life not be extended by life-sustaining procedures, including the administration of nutrition and hydration artificially.

_____ I direct that my life not be extended by life-sustaining procedures, except that if I am unable to take food and water by mouth, I wish to receive nutrition and hydration artificially.

4. _____ I direct that, no matter what my condition, medication to relieve pain and suffering not be given to me if the medication would shorten my remaining life.

5. _____ I direct that, no matter what my condition, I be given all available medical treatment in accordance with accepted health care standards.

Advance Directive Part B (continued)

6. If I am pregnant, my decision concerning life-sustaining procedures shall be modified as follows:

_____
_____
_____
_____

7. I direct (in the following space, indicate any other instructions regarding receipt or non-receipt of any health care): _____

_____
_____
_____

By signing below, I indicate that I am emotionally and mentally competent to make this Advance Directive and that I understand its purpose and effect of this document.

_____   _____
(Date)   (Signature of Declarant)

The declarant signed or acknowledged signing these health care instructions in my presence and, based upon my personal observation, appears to be a competent individual,

_____   _____
(Witness)   (Witness)

_____   _____
_____   _____
_____   _____

(Signature and addresses of Two Witnesses)

Organic Donation Addendum

[Note: If you want to be an organ donor, you can attach this page to your living will or advance directive. Sign it and have it witnessed.]

Upon my death, I wish to donate:
_____ Any needed organs, tissues, or eyes.
_____ Only the following organs, tissues, or eyes:

_____
_____
_____

I authorize the use of my organs, tissues, or eyes:
_____ for transplantation;
_____ for therapy;
_____ for research;
_____ for medical education;
_____ for any purpose authorized by law.

I understand that before any vital organ, tissue, or eye may be removed for transplantation, I must be pronounced dead. After death, I direct that all support measures be continued to maintain the viability for transplantation of my organs, tissues, and eyes until organ, tissue and eye recovery has been completed.

I understand that my estate will not be charged for any costs associated with my decision to donate my organs, tissues, or eyes or the actual disposition on my organs, tissues, or eyes.

By signing below, I indicate that I am emotionally and mentally competent to make this organ donation addendum and that I understand its purpose and effect of this document.

_____   _____
(Date)   (Signature of Declarant)

The declarant signed or acknowledged signing this organ donation addendum in my presence and, based upon my personal observation, appears to be a competent individual.

_____   _____
(Witness)   (Witness)

(Signature two Witnesses)

Organic Donation Addendum

[Note: If you want to be an organ donor, you can attach this page to your living will or advance directive. Sign it and have it witnessed.]

Upon my death, I wish to donate:

_____ Any needed organs, tissues, or eyes.

_____ Only the following organs, tissues, or eyes:

_____

_____

_____

I authorize the use of my organs, tissues, or eyes:

_____ for transplantation;

_____ for therapy;

_____ for research;

_____ for medical education;

_____ for any purpose authorized by law.

I understand that before any vital organ, tissue, or eye may be removed for transplantation, I must be pronounced dead. After death, I direct that all support measures be continued to maintain the viability for transplantation of my organs, tissues, and eyes until organ, tissue and eye recovery has been completed.

I understand that my estate will not be charged for any costs associated with my decision to donate my organs, tissues, or eyes or the actual disposition on my organs, tissues, or eyes.

By signing below, I indicate that I am emotionally and mentally competent to make this organ donation addendum and that I understand its purpose and effect of this document.

_____   _____
(Date)   (Signature of Declarant)

The declarant signed or acknowledged signing this organ donation addendum in my presence and, based upon my personal observation, appears to be a competent individual.

_____   _____
(Witness)   (Witness)

(Signature two Witnesses)

Do-Not-Resuscinate Order

I request that in the event my heart and breathing should stop, no person shall attempt to resuscitate me.

This order is effective until it is revoked by me.

Being of sound mind, I voluntarily execute this order, and I understand it's full import.

_____

(Declarant's signature and date)

_____

(Type or print declarant's full name)

_____

(Signature of person who signed for declarant, if applicable and date)

_____

(Type or print full name)

Attestation of Witnesses

The individual who has executed this order appears to ne of sound mind, and under no duress, fraud, or undue influence. Upon executing this order, the individual has (has not) received an identification bracelet.

_____

(Witness signature and date)

_____

(Type or print witness's name)

_____

(Witness signature and date)

_____

(Type or print witness's name)

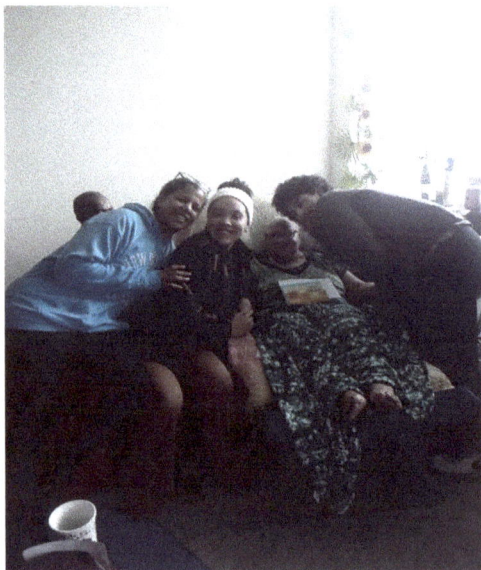

Avel with friends of the family. Left to right, Tricia, Ebonie, Avel, Aidan

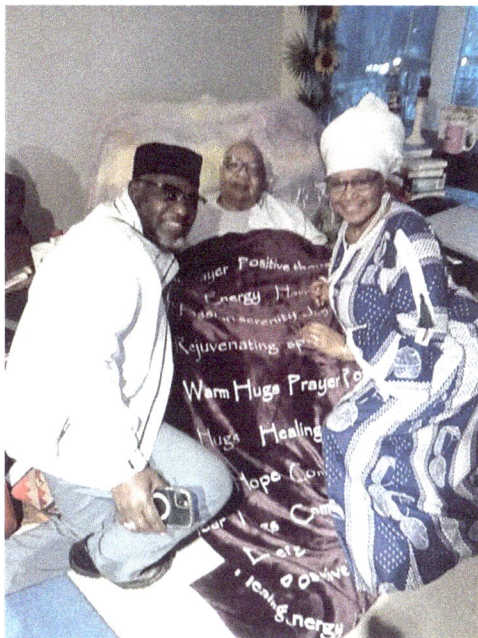

Mikal Shabazz and Shafia Monroe Shabazz hanging out
with Senator Avel Gordly middle of photo

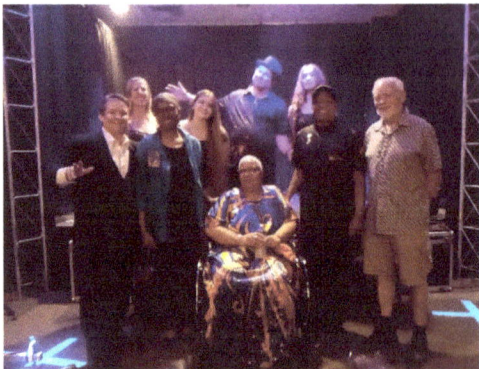

Senator Avel Gordly at a neighborhood magic show activity with All American Magic Shop and Theatre cast and crew front row left to right Mark Benthimer (Magician Owner All American Magic) (friend) Gloria Gostnell, Senator Avel Gordly, (Son) Tyrone Waters, (friend) David Gostnell

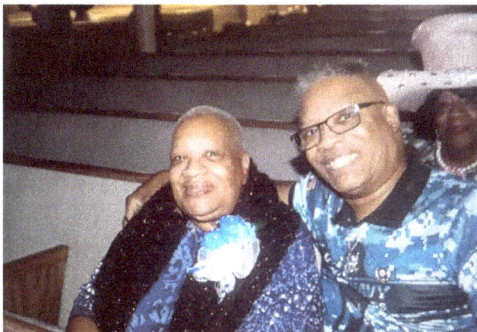

Attending Highland Christian Center for spiritual enrichment Left to right Senator Avel Gordly (Son) Tyrone Waters Second row Church Mother Nancy Smith.

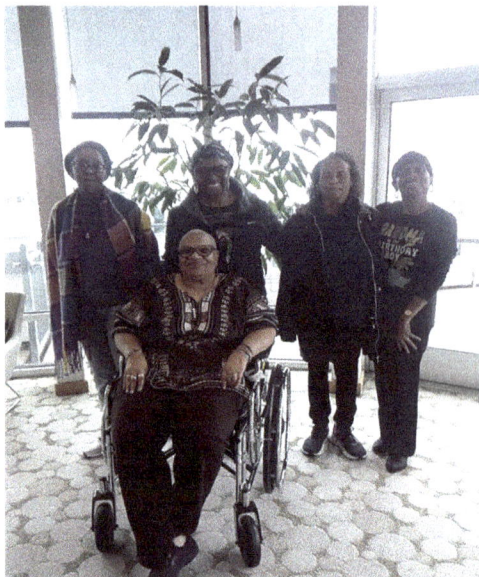

Hanging out with reading group Front row Senator Avel Gordly Second row left to right Karen Powell, Gloria Gostnell, Emily Bates, Bev Johnson.

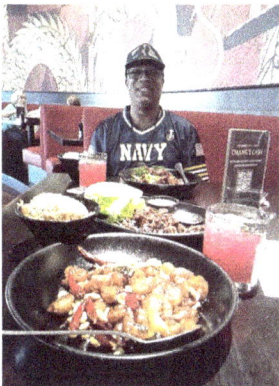

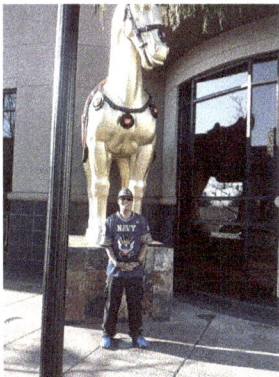

Rev. Dr. Tyrone W. Waters Taking care of himself having personal respite time lunch at a local restaurant in Lake Oswego, Oregon.

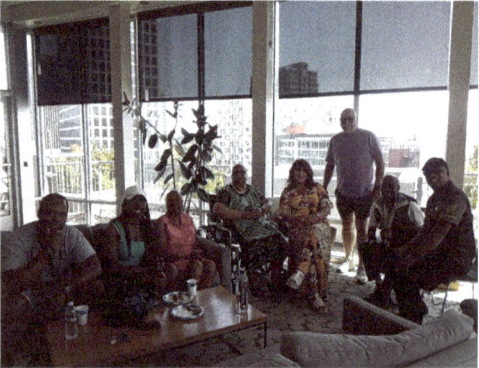

Senator Avel Gordly hanging out with family, left to right,
Thabiti, Rashonda, Anita, Avel, Tina, Michael, Brian,
Tyrone, not pictured Eqwe, Nashid.

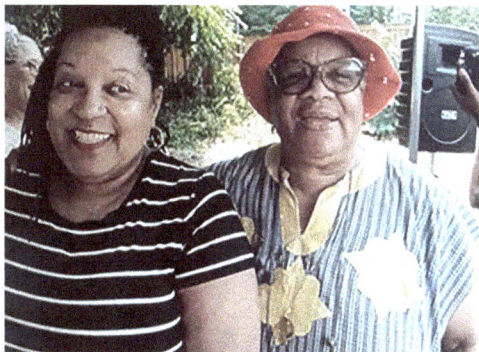

Avel with her sister, Faye.

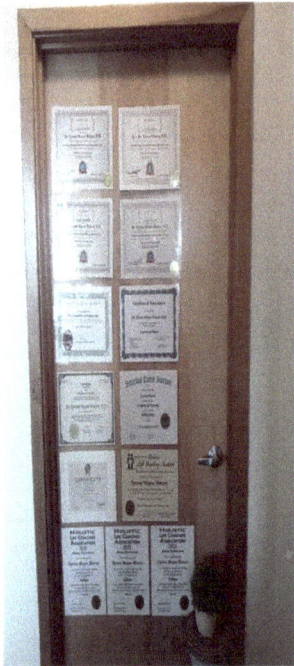

Rev. Dr. Tyrone W. Waters academic accomplishments

www.ingramcontent.com/pod-product-compliance
Lightning Source LLC
Chambersburg PA
CBHW040849210326
41597CB00029B/4783